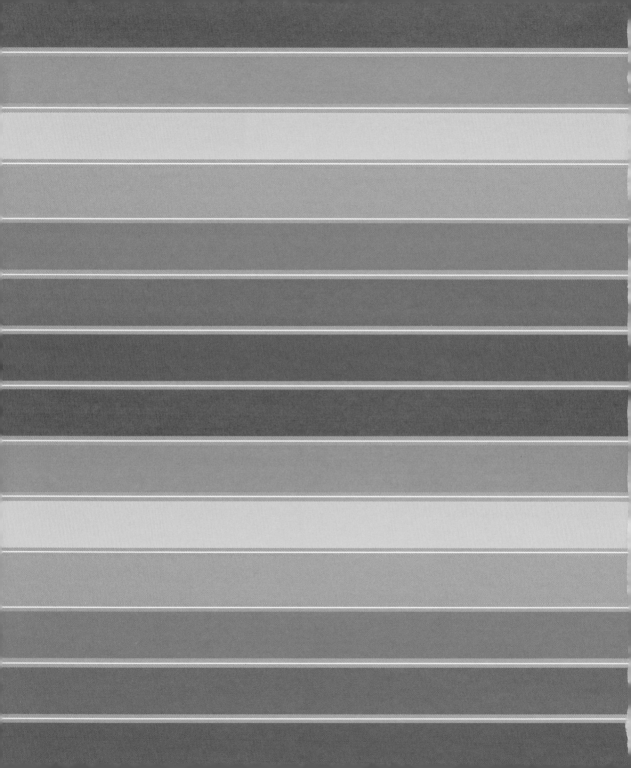

"*The Rainbow Juice Cleanse* provides a path to a life free of sugar addiction and unhealthy eating habits. Following this seven-day juice cleanse will give you access to more energy, clearer skin, a slimmer waistline, and the tools you need to continue discovering your healthiest self."

—Vani Hari, activist, founder of FoodBabe.com, and author of *The Food Babe Way*

"Dr. Ginger's rainbow approach to juice cleansing is so unique and comprehensive. She offers accessible information and delicious recipes that will help you reclaim your health and have fun!"

—Tess Masters, author of *The Blender Girl*

"*The Rainbow Juice Cleanse* is a revolutionary program that utilizes the incredible benefits of phytonutrients to support weight loss and detox, and is an important book in today's unhealthy Standard American Diet world."

—Danielle Omar, MS, RDN, author of *Skinny Juices*

"Today's confusing field of nutrition can paralyze a health seeker's progress. Dr. Ginger's Rainbow Juice Cleanse will clarify, guide, and comprehensively lead the reader into maximum health and happiness."

—Brian Clement, PhD, NMD, LN, international speaker, author, and co-director of the Hippocrates Health Institute

"While most eat their way to premature aging with processed fast food, Dr. Ginger shows us it is possible to control much of your own aging in *The Rainbow Juice Cleanse*. If you want great skin, a lean body, and longevity consider this book your repair kit."

—Robert M. Goldman, MD, PhD, DO, FAASP, co-founder and chairman of the A4M (American Academy of Anti-Aging Medicine)

"With lots of detailed information and tasty recipes, along with beautiful photos, Dr. Ginger shows you how to achieve your highest level of health by eating the colors of the rainbow."

—Robert Cheeke, bestselling author of *Vegan Bodybuilding & Fitness* and *Shred It!*

"If you've ever had any doubts about the benefits of juicing, they'll disappear after reading this book! *The Rainbow Juice Cleanse* goes into detail about why, what, and how we should juice, and explains the importance of eating our fruit and drinking our veggies. It's my new go-to bible for all things juicing-related."

—Andrea Donsky, RHN, author of *Unjunk Your Junk Food* and radio host of *Naturally Savvy Radio* on RadioMD.com

"The most potent drugs my patients can take are the foods they choose to consume. Dr. Ginger gives you great insight into the healing you can receive from *The Rainbow Juice Cleanse*."

—Ray D. Strand, MD, bestselling author of *Healthy for Life* and *What Your Doctor Doesn't Know About Nutritional Medicine May Be Killing You*

THE RAINBOW
JUICE CLEANSE

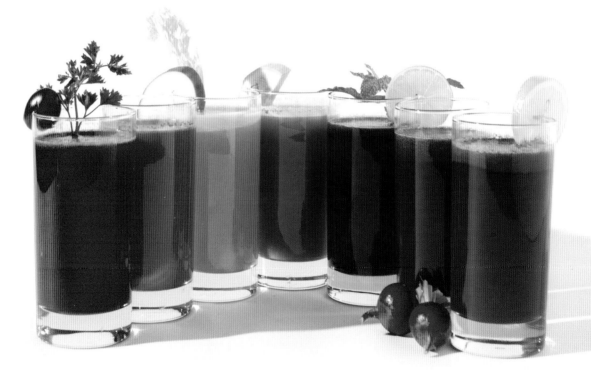

THE RAINBOW
JUICE CLEANSE

Lose Weight, Boost Energy, and
Supercharge Your Health

DR. GINGER SOUTHALL

RUNNING PRESS
PHILADELPHIA • LONDON

© 2015 by Dr. Ginger Southall
Photography © 2015 by Allan Penn
A Hollan Publishing, Inc. Concept

Recipe on page 113 is printed with permission from the Hippocrates Health Institute.

Published by Running Press,
A Member of the Perseus Books Group

Books published by Running Press are available at special discounts for bulk purchases in the United States by corporations, institutions, and other organizations. For more information, please contact the Special Markets Department at the Perseus Books Group, 2300 Chestnut Street, Suite 200, Philadelphia, PA 19103, or call (800) 810-4145, ext. 5000, or e-mail special.markets@perseusbooks.com.

ISBN 978-0-7624-5734-2
Library of Congress Control Number: 2014951438

E-book ISBN 978-0-7624-5738-0

9 8 7 6 5 4 3 2
Digit on the right indicates the number of this printing

Cover and interior design by Susan Van Horn
Edited by Jordana Tusman
Typography: Brandon Text, Garage Gothic, and Reverie

Running Press Book Publishers
2300 Chestnut Street
Philadelphia, PA 19103-4371

Visit us on the web!
www.offthemenublog.com
www.runningpress.com

FOR MY MOTHER, KAY—

my shining example of love, grace, strength,
sacrifice, and godly womanhood.
May this book be the impetus you need to finally
open that box I bought you with the word *juicer*
on it and start juicing once and for all!
Love you more.

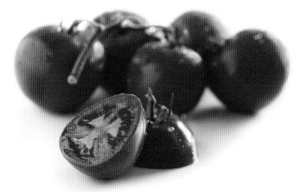

CONTENTS

"Eat your fruit;
  juice your veggies."

—DR. GINGER

WHAT'S UP WITH JUICING?

EVEN IF YOU ARE NOT FAMILIAR WITH THE CONCEPT of "juicing," you can't own a television and not have heard of Jack LaLanne. For years on end, his infomercials about his Jack LaLanne Power Juicer aired at all hours of the day and night. He was still going strong late into his nineties and attributed his great health to decades of consistent juicing and exercising.

But juicing isn't something new. In fact, it is a practice that dates back to the ancient cultures of the world. In the biblical era, juices for healing were promoted by the Essenes in the Dead Sea Scrolls. In ancient India, Ayrevedic practitioners utilized various "pressed" herbs and vegetables, as well as consuming various fruits for healing purposes. The healing powers of juices and other foods have been recognized for centuries. But foods have not become part of mainstream healing in the Western world, even though Hippocrates, the ancient Greek physician and the father of modern medicine, famously said, "Let food be thy medicine and medicine be thy food."

Over the past century, many have blazed the juicing trail under the mainstream radar. Dr. Max Gerson (author of *A Cancer Therapy*) is said to have healed both himself and others suffering from ailments as diverse as migraines, diabetes, and cancer with juicing. Dr. Norman W. Walker (and his Walker Press Juicer),

Patricia Bragg and Paul C. Bragg (authors of *Bragg Healthy Lifestyle*), Jay Kordich (author of *The Juiceman's Power of Juicing*), Ann Wigmore (author of *The Wheatgrass Book*), Kris Carr (author of the *Crazy Sexy Cancer* book series), and the directors of the Hippocrates Health Institute, Drs. Brian and Anna Maria Clement (who have made raw green juices a staple of the nutritional protocol for their guests) have all put their own "squeeze" on the healing powers of juicing. Political leaders, clergy, athletes, supermodels, and, more recently, cancer survivors and talk show hosts like Dr. Mehmet Oz have all made a significant impact by helping others learn about the power of juicing.

As I progressed through my own career as a health and healing expert and passionately learned and witnessed firsthand how juices and "real" food can radically transform one's health, weight, family, and entire life, I decided to make a conscious choice to look at everything I eat and drink from a healing mind-set. And that's how the idea for this book began. Today, you can find hundreds of books on juicing. There are juice shops on every corner, it seems, and a juicing infomercial airing every hour on television. But the frustrating part, from a true healing perspective, is that many of them are missing a crucial component.

The Rainbow Juice Cleanse boldly revamps the entire thought process behind the popular juicing trend because it is written from the perspective of how juicing fruit and a few popular high-glycemic vegetables affect the intricate physiology of the body. Weight loss, detoxification, and even reversing the progress of disease cannot take place without this basic understanding, but sadly most popular juicing books neglect to address it.

If you want to lose weight and detoxify your body, if you have diabetes or any type of blood-sugar issue, or even if you have a disease like cancer—you should not be juicing fruit. Juiced fruit is basically a glass of sugar, and yet fruit is usually the major component—and sometimes the only component—in almost all the recipes in the popular juicing books and juice bars

> Juicing fruit and a few popular high-glycemic vegetables affect the intricate physiology of the body.

out there, because we, as a society, are all addicted to sugar.

In my health seminars and my private sessions with clients, when it comes to juicing, I always say, "Eat your fruit; juice your veggies." In this book you will learn why.

The Rainbow Juice Cleanse is a revolutionary program that employs the nutritious, slimming, and healing properties of juicing delicious vegetables, not fruit, to kick-start weight loss and improve health. In just seven days, you will begin to detoxify your body and lose up to seven pounds! Each day of the program focuses on a different color of the rainbow, utilizing savory veggies and detoxifying herbs and spices you may never have thought of juicing, as well as Rainbow boosts you can add to your juice (pages 62-65), ensuring the best possible nutritional profile and guaranteeing positive results.

This book will teach you how to choose the right juicer, properly shop the rainbow of nutritious, alkaline produce that Mother Nature provides, and avoid the common pitfalls and ticking sugar bombs that we often ignore, to the detriment of our health. It guides you on how to "drink the rainbow" with a plan that entails consuming phytonutrient-rich, colorful juices and drinking a different color each day of the cleanse. It then shows you how to reach your pot of gold at the end of the rainbow after just seven days. It's a jump start on losing weight, detoxifying your body, countering the effects of aging, gaining abundant energy, reversing the progress of disease, and balancing your body and its pH overall.

For those who have never tried a juice cleanse before, two options are offered before you transition into the juice-only, seven-day Rainbow Juice Cleanse.

The first option is a two-week program called the Rainbow Warm-Up, during which you continue with your regular diet (with some major encouragement to give some Rainbow food recipes a try), and you also

> The Rainbow Juice Cleanse is a revolutionary program that employs the nutritious, slimming, and healing properties of juicing delicious vegetables, not fruit, to kick-start weight loss and improve health.

start incorporating one Rainbow Cleanse juice per day into your diet.

The second option is the one-week Rainbow Rev-Up, during which you consume one juice per day (or more if you like), and consume only the Rainbow foods and the Rainbow food recipes. With this approach, you do away with all your unhealthy food habits and no longer follow the Standard American Diet (SAD)—a highly appropriate acronym, don't you think? For one day a week during the Rainbow Rev-Up phase, you will consume only juice the entire day—as much as you want—a little taste, if you will, of what to expect during the full seven-day Rainbow Juice Cleanse.

You may choose to start with the warm-up and then ease into the rev-up, or you may be feeling braver and start with the rev-up and then proceed to the Rainbow Juice Cleanse. Or, you may just want to skip both beginner phases altogether and jump right into the juice-only Rainbow Cleanse. Any one of these options is fine— do what works for you!

But when you move on to the juice-only, seven-day Rainbow Juice Cleanse, the Rainbow rewards really kick into high gear. For four days before and four days after the cleanse, you will eat very easily digestible foods from the Rainbow foods list as you ease into and then ease out of the juice cleanse.

OK, are you ready? You're about to turn into a rainbow juicing trailblazer in your own home and community. Let's go; let's learn; let's juice!

PART 1
THE RAINBOW EXPLAINED

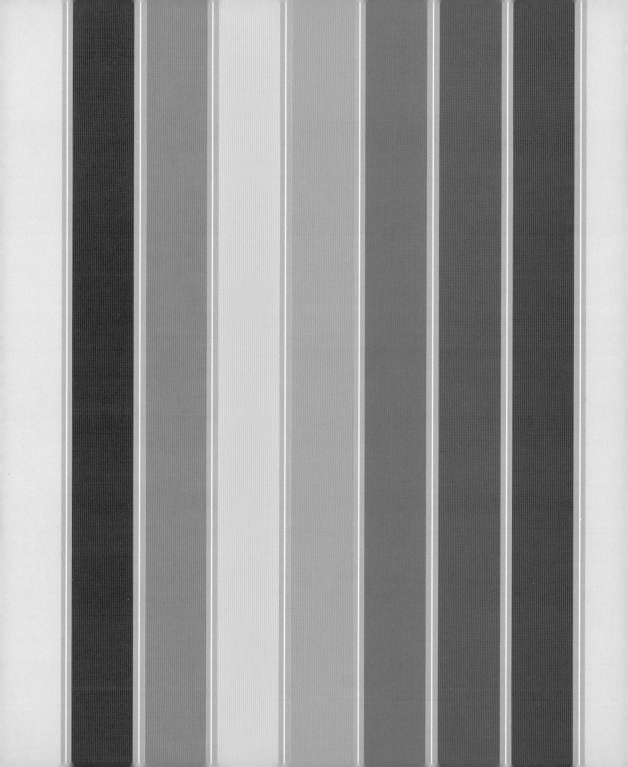

1

WHY THE RAINBOW?

ALTHOUGH SIR ISAAC NEWTON WAS THE FIRST to understand the rainbow from a scientific perspective, for centuries, in many cultures, there have been countless myths and legends surrounding their power. The rainbow has historically been a symbol of hope, faith, and the promise of a brighter future ahead.

I even have memories of childhood elders saying, "Eat the colors of the rainbow, and you will allow the sunlight to shine through you," or "Eat the colors of the rainbow and watch your life explode with beauty and color."

As an adult and a physician who has extensively studied food, nutrition, disease, and the human body, I can say that both the symbolism and the childhood sayings ring true. Eating the foods of the colors of the rainbow—red, orange, yellow, green, blue, indigo, and violet—indeed *can* lead to the promise of a brighter future for both our weight and our overall health.

● Why Color?

One word: *phytonutrients*.

Nature's naturally colored plant foods—with their vibrant red, orange, yellow, green, and other bright colors—contain phytonutrients (also known as phytochemicals). These are classes of active plant chemicals that offer above and beyond the basic vitamins and minerals, fats, proteins, and carbs, and supercharge our health. There are tens of thousands of phytonutrients in nature's foods, and each is known to have a different and very potent biological effect. Phytonutrients are said to protect the body from a wide array of illnesses and modern diseases, such as cancer, diabetes, heart disease, high blood pressure, stroke, and other serious health challenges. In addition, some enhance immunity; some are anti-inflammatory; some work as potent antioxidants and even repair DNA; and some are fat-burning and anti-aging powerhouses.

You may already be familiar with phytonutrients and not realize it. One of the best-known families of phytonutrients are the carotenoids, of which there are over six hundred. Beta-carotene, found in carrots and recognized for being good for the eyes, is the most familiar. But nature abounds in phytonutrients, many of which have yet to be discovered. Scientists are continuing to unmask more and more benefits of these amazing health boosters and their transformative effects on the body.

● Count Colors, Not Calories

Nature's foods of the same color do not necessarily contain the exact same vitamins, minerals, or phytonutrients, but many do share predominant phytonutrients. Oftentimes, the phytonutrient gives the produce its vibrant color. So clustering colors together, as the Rainbow Juice Cleanse does, not only loads the body with essential vitamins and minerals, but also supercharges it with the dominant phytonutrients (and there are lots of them) of that color. Keep in mind that it's not about eating just two or three superfoods; it's about consuming a diet comprising a wide array of colorful plant foods on a daily basis because they are all super for health, vitality, cleansing, and weight loss. Most of us don't consume enough fruits and veggies on a daily basis, which means most of us don't consume enough phytonutrients. In fact, 76 percent of us are not getting enough of them in our diet; that's eight out of ten Americans shortchanging themselves of these vital nutrients. Clustering colors creates a fun way to remind us that colors equal health. By consuming a different color each day, you will be sure to get all the colors of the rainbow in just seven days.

THE COLOR GROUPS

Below are the colors we use for the Rainbow Juice Cleanse with some of their most important phytonutrients, benefits, and the foods where they're found listed for each one, as well as the percentage of American adults not consuming adequate amounts of these life- and health-giving nutrients.

RED

PHYTONUTRIENTS:

- Lycopene
- Carotenoids
- Ellagic acid
- Quercetin
- Hesperidin
- Anthocyanins

BENEFITS:

- Supports urinary tract, prostate, and DNA health
- Protects against heart disease and cancer

FOUND IN:

- Tomatoes
- Raspberries
- Red cabbage
- Cranberries
- Red peppers

74% fall short

ORANGE

PHYTONUTRIENTS:

- Alpha-carotene
- Beta-carotene
- Beta-cryptoxanthin

BENEFITS:

- Supports eye health, healthy immune function, and overall health, growth, and development

FOUND IN:

- Carrots
- Orange peppers
- Sweet potatoes
- Pumpkin
- Turmeric
- Ginger

80% fall short

YELLOW

PHYTONUTRIENTS:

- Lutein
- Zeaxanthin

BENEFITS:

- Supports retinal and overall eye health

FOUND IN:

- Spaghetti squash
- Yellow peppers
- Lemons
- Pineapple

80% fall short

GREEN

PHYTONUTRIENTS:

- Sulforaphane
- Chlorophyll
- Indoles
- Lutein
- EGCG (epigallocatechin gallate)
- Isothiocyanate
- Isoflavones

BENEFITS:

- Supports artery function, liver function, eye health, and cell health
- Promotes gum health and wound healing
- Keeps bones and teeth strong

FOUND IN:

- Leafy greens
- Sprouted grasses and algae
- Cucumber
- Zucchini
- Peas
- Avocado
- Asparagus

69% fall short

BLUE/INDIGO/VIOLET

PHYTONUTRIENTS:

- Resveratrol
- Flavonoids
- Anthocyanins

BENEFITS:

- Supports brain, bone, heart, and artery health
- Boosts memory
- Protects against cancer
- Counters aging

FOUND IN:

- Purple cabbage
- Blueberries
- Blackberries
- Eggplant
- Beets

75% fall short

WHITE/TAN/BROWN

PHYTONUTRIENTS:

- Allicin
- Sulfides
- Anthoxanthins

BENEFITS:

- Anticancer and anti-inflammatory properties, boosts immunity, helps to lower blood pressure and cholesterol

FOUND IN:

- Garlic
- Onions
- Scallions
- Cauliflower
- Bananas
- Mushrooms
- Ginger

83% fall short

NOTE: Although not among the colors of the rainbow, white/tan/brown and their corresponding foods have many incredible health benefits and are found in the Rainbow Juice Cleanse recipes.

●Slimming Colors

The Rainbow Juice Cleanse strips away pounds, eliminates nasty toxins, and slows down the aging process by establishing the right environment in the body for natural and sustained weight loss, detoxification, and anti-aging. In addition, it promotes great health overall. The cleanse accomplishes this in several ways.

PHYTONUTRIENTS

More and more studies are showing that phytonutrients aid in weight loss. A study published in a 2008 issue of the *Journal of Agricultural and Food Chemistry* shows that the class of phytonutrients called anthocyanins helps stimulate the fat-burning process and significantly counters obesity. Another study in the November–December 2010 issue of *Biofactors* found that phytochemicals, particularly flavonoids, potentially inhibit the transformation of the fat cells' precursor cells into actual fat cells. They also stimulate the breakdown of fats and thereby reduce the girth of the amount of overall fat tissue. Many other phytonutrients of different families have similar effects. This means that consuming large quantities of phytonutrients, as we do in the Rainbow Juice Cleanse, will help promote weight loss.

> Phytonutrients will help promote weight loss.

ALKALINITY, HYDRATION, AND DETOXIFICATION

Remember high school chemistry and the pH scale? Believe it or not, the pH scale has important implications for both health and weight loss. If you recall, the scale runs from 0 to 14, with 7 being neutral. The numbers below 7 are considered acidic and those above 7 are considered alkaline. Your body likes to be just slightly alkaline, at a pH of about 7.36–7.45, and it can be if you consume nature's foods in their least processed form. Unfortunately, most of us are very acidic and dehydrated, due to an unhealthy lifestyle involving stress, no exercise, and consumption of highly cooked and highly acidic foods, such as coffee, alcohol, processed meats, fried foods, chips, ice cream, sodas, and artificial sweeteners. This kind of lifestyle makes the body very acidic, which is the ideal breeding ground for disease. In this acidic state, you also store in your fat cells all the acids and toxins you consume, making it very difficult for you to lose weight. Consuming hydrating, detoxifying, alkaline produce, as we do in the Rainbow Juice Cleanse, allows the body to release toxic weight easily and safely.

CONSUMING THE RIGHT SUGARS AND BLOOD SUGAR STABILIZATION

The type of sugars we consume and our blood sugar levels throughout the day determine whether we store the food we eat as fat or burn it as energy. We will learn more about this in chapter 2. The trick to losing weight and keeping it all off are to consume foods with what's called a low glycemic index (GI) throughout the day and to consume the *right* types of sugars, as we do in the Rainbow Juice Cleanse. This keeps your blood sugar on an even keel.

The Rainbow Juice Cleanse juices and the Rainbow Juice Cleanse foods are all loaded with very hydrating, alkaline, lower-glycemic, fat-busting phytonutrients, as well as vitamins, minerals, amino acids, enzymes, oxygen, and organic water, creating an absolutely perfect environment for massive detoxification, incredible nourishment, and subsequent weight loss to occur in a short period.

So, let's get started exploring the rainbow and the pot of gold that awaits you at its end!

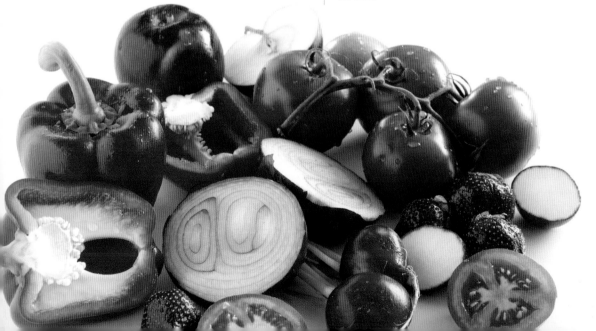

CHAPTER

PITFALLS TO FINDING THE TREASURE AT THE END OF THE RAINBOW

LET'S TALK ABOUT some of the pitfalls, speed bumps, and traps you may fall into during the Rainbow Juice Cleanse program.

Juices versus Smoothies versus Shakes

When you first learn about juicing, you might confuse a juice with a smoothie or a shake. It's important to differentiate among these because, from a healing perspective, each one has particular health benefits associated with it. I recommend incorporating all three into your regular diet over time. Everyone seems to have a different definition, so here is how I define each in my recipes.

JUICES

Fresh-made juices are made in a juicer, which extracts the juice from the fibrous pulp, providing massive amounts of hydrating and highly absorbable organic water and a concentrated form of naturally occurring vitamins, minerals, chlorophyll, phytochemicals, and enzymes. This delivers more nutrition than you could ever eat in the form of solid food in one sitting. It is important to make your juices fresh and to use *only* organic produce. Store-bought, pasteurized, processed, or refined juices are not comparable, for these have added processed salt, sugar and/or artificial sweeteners, artificial colors, so-called "natural flavors," and toxic preservatives. In addition, many have been "enriched" with synthetic chemical nutrients and other unwanted additives.

Juices are great for pregnant and nursing mothers; for people with cancer, HIV, or other conditions where the immune system is too compromised to extract nutrients from food; and for anyone desiring energy and a quick "boost." Juices are also great for those seeking to lose toxic weight; for, there is no digestive energy expended here, so your body can focus on cleansing and nourishing, which is what we want during our seven-day cleanse. Juices are absorbed almost instantly; they give you immediate energy; and they are pure liquid nutrition! And, as you will learn, when I say *juice*, I mean veggie juice, not fruit juice.

> It is important to make your juices fresh and to use only organic produce.

SMOOTHIES

You're sure to get your daily dose of fiber and more in a cool, refreshing smoothie. Unlike juices, smoothies are made by tossing the entire vegetable into a high-speed blender (along with filtered water), which keeps the fiber in the final product. Fiber acts like a magic sponge that pulls out toxic wastes—and even cholesterol—from our bodies. So smoothies are an excellent, natural way to lower high cholesterol. This is where I give you a little more leeway in consuming fruit, although I still want to remind you of my mantra: *Eat your fruit; juice your veggies.* If you incorporate fruit in your smoothie, make it less than 10 percent of your total daily calorie intake. Smoothies give you a feeling of fullness, more so than juices, due to their massive amounts of fiber. Refreshing, filling, energy-giving, and addictive, a smoothie works well as a snack or a meal substitute.

SHAKES

Shakes are a great way to add healthy plant-based proteins (yes, plants do have protein!) and the good-for-you fats to your diet without any of the chemical additives found in commercial "muscle building" formulas. No hormones, steroids, antibiotics, or cholesterol in these "milk" shakes; just dairy-free, creamy-blended nuts, seeds, or sprouted grains, chock-full of highly absorbable protein, vitamin E, bioavailable calcium, great flavor, and the good fats your body needs. Got nut milk?

● What Is a Fruit?
What Is a Veggie?

The infamous debate—Is it a fruit or a vegetable?—has pervaded society and even the courts as far back as the 1800s. In 1893, the law actually had to step in to decide a case regarding tomatoes, thus perhaps fueling our confusion today on the tomato's proper designation.

Nix v. Hedden, a U.S. Supreme Court case, resulted in a unanimous ruling that imported tomatoes should indeed be taxed as vegetables and not as fruits, which, at the time, were taxed at a lower rate. The High Court drew on the "ordinary" kitchen definitions of fruits and vegetables to define a tomato, although the justices did concede that a tomato, botanically speaking, is classified as a fruit.

You may think you've known since you were five years old how to differentiate a fruit from a vegetable, but unless you are a gardener or a chef or a lawmaker, your view may fall somewhere in between.

According to the study of plants (botany), a fruit is the sweet and fleshy product of a tree or other plant that contains seeds. All the other parts of the plant—the leaves, stems, and roots—are considered vegetables.

By that definition, gardeners would define avocados, cucumbers, squash, and tomatoes as fruits. By contrast, leafy plants, such as lettuce, spinach, and kale; and stem plants, such as broccoli and celery; and root plants, such as beets, potatoes, and jicama would all be categorized as vegetables.

From a culinary perspective, however, the definition is more nuanced. Foods that may be botanically considered fruits, but which taste less sweet and more savory, are considered vegetables by the culinary world. So chefs would classify botanical fruits, such as bell peppers, eggplants, and tomatoes, as vegetables.

In the Rainbow Juice Cleanse, we generally follow the chef's definition of fruits and veggies, and consider bell peppers, cucumbers, avocados, and tomatoes as vegetables. But, more importantly, we look at them from another perspective: the weight loss, cleansing, and healing perspective. In doing that, we take into account three important factors.

TOXICITY TO THE BODY

We know fruits and veggies, in general, are not toxic to the body, although there are a few specific health challenges that call for avoiding certain produce until the condition is under control. What I'm referring to here is pesticides, herbicides, and fungicides. In the Rainbow Juice Cleanse, the foods, recipes, and particularly the juices should incorporate only organic or chemical-free produce. This is a cleanse, and your body absorbs these juices immediately without the usual sequence of processing, so you want to keep your body totally free of dangerous and potentially cancer-causing substances.

GLYCEMIC INDEX/LOAD AND TYPE OF SUGAR

The glycemic index (GI) is a measure of how fast and how high your blood sugar rises (and then falls) after you have eaten a carbohydrate-rich (especially sugary) food. For example, white sugar has a GI of 100, which is very high. This is the standard against which all other foods are measured. The scale runs from 0 to 100.

Low GI value = *55 or less*
Intermediate GI value = *56–69*
High GI value = *70 or more*

The GI value of a baked potato is 85, a Cookies and Cream Clif Builder's Bar is 101, and orange-flavored Gatorade is 89. On the other hand, an avocado, cauliflower, celery, cucumber, leafy veggies (spinach, kale), and nuts all have a GI value of 0. Fruits have higher GI values, as do certain veggies, such as carrots (47) and beets (64).

Eating fruits and higher-glycemic vegetables should cause no problems; whole carrots, beets, and all fruits are on the Rainbow Juice Cleanse foods list. When you eat them whole, their overall glycemic impact is negligible, for the most part, but I still recommend keeping them at about 10 percent or less of your total calorie intake.

Why? Because, most likely, your diet has always revolved around a sea of sugar, and we are here to get that under control.

When you start juicing the high-glycemic fruits and veggies (keep in mind that you can juice an entire bag of carrots and fill just one glass of juice), this can become a problem, especially for sugar-sensitive individuals. (And remember: I'm coming at this entire program from a healing perspective.) Lower-GI foods keep insulin levels low; thus, by consuming these foods you won't stimulate fat storage, and you'll maximize weight loss.

The other key feature to consider is the fructose content, which is the main type of sugar in fruits and root veggies. Oddly enough, fructose doesn't raise blood sugar, as you would expect. But what it does do, which you will learn later in this chapter, is turn into fat. Ugh! And we are *not* interested in that happening during this cleanse.

Remember my rule: *Eat your fruit; juice your veggies* (except carrots and beets).

Now here is where it gets tricky and why the GI value (or even the GI load, another measurement that considers the

> Fructose doesn't raise blood sugar, but it does turn to fat.

food serving sizes) is not the best or the only factor to look at in your overall diet. A hot dog has a lower GI value than a pineapple, but I would *never* recommend eating a hot dog or feeding one to your kids, or even your dog, for that matter!

PHYTONUTRIENT AND OVERALL MICRONUTRIENT CONTENT

Although the GI has been scientifically validated as a tool in helping to control conditions such as diabetes, and has been around since about 1981, it can't be used in isolation. You have to look at other key factors during the cleanse and its warm-up and rev-up phases. You need to consider the overall phytonutrient and micronutrient content in what you consume.

All the foods and juices in the program are so alkaline, nutritionally dense, and jam-packed with phytonutrients, they innately give off the following side effects: They decrease previously uncontrollable food cravings; they speed up weight loss and cleansing; and they harness incredible disease-protective qualities. And who doesn't want all that?

● The World of Sugar

A major tenet in this program is under-standing sugar—how it affects your brain, how it creates chaos in your body, how the different types are broken down and used by the body, how it relates to disease, and how it impedes your weight loss and cleansing journey. So it's important to get some cru-cial background information. I promise you will have a brand-new view of sugar, in all its deceptive forms, by the end of this chapter. Let's first tackle the sugar producers.

THE SUGAR INDUSTRY

The sugar industry is a multibillion-dollar business, supported by substantial govern-ment subsidies. Today it is receiving its fair share of criticism from those who think the U.S. sugar policy artificially inflates sugar prices to benefit the sugar producers at the expense of consumer health. Many are also saying Big Sugar has become the new tobacco, deploying some of the same tactics used by Big Tobacco decades ago to downplay and misrepresent that too much of a sweet thing can be a very dan-gerous thing to your health and longevity.

THE SUGAR RUSH

In the nineteenth century, only the aris-tocracy and the most affluent in the com-munity consumed processed sugar—it was almost like a delicacy. Ironically, today's sugar subsidies have the poorest mem-bers of our society consuming the largest amount of sugar, because so many of the foods made with it are so cheap. Today, sugar has become such a staple in the aver-age American diet that many people are completely unaware of how much of it they are actually consuming. But let me start by saying we eat 75,000 percent more sugar than our ancestors did. Yikes!

According to the U.S. Department of Agriculture (USDA), the United States is the world's largest consumer of sweeten-ers, one of the largest sugar producers, as well as one of the largest producers of sugarcane and sugar beets, particularly from Florida and Louisiana.

The worldwide consumption of sugar continues to rise every year. According to George Washington University's Face the Facts project, on average, American adults consume almost thirty teaspoons

> We eat 75,000 percent more sugar than our ancestors did.

(150 ml) of the sweet stuff per day (almost five hundred calories); that's one hundred pounds (45.5 kg) of sugar and sweeteners each year, and nearly half of that, they say, comes from carbonated sodas and fruit drinks. The American Heart Association recommends consuming no more than six teaspoons (30 ml) per day (one hundred calories).

Since 1990, the World Health Organization (WHO) has advised that intake of free sugars should be less than 10 percent of total energy (calorie) intake per day. "Free sugars" are sugars that are added to foods by the manufacturer, the cook, or the consumer. The term *free sugars* also encompasses honey, fruit concentrates, and processed fruit juices.

The WHO further notes that reducing the intake of sugar to below 5 percent would have additional benefits. Five percent of overall calorie intake would equal about six teaspoons (30 ml) of sugar per day for an adult. Keep in mind that one tablespoon (15 ml) of regular ketchup contains one teaspoon (5 ml) of sugar (5 ml) and a can of soda contains ten teaspoons (50 ml) of sugar. So with today's Standard American Diet, someone would be hard-pressed to meet these suggested guidelines, much less the older ones.

One hundred pounds (45.5 kg) of sugar—our current average annual intake—certainly translates into a lot of additional weight in one year. Is it surprising that obesity and so many other diseases have become such dominant health issues?

● What's in a Name?

In order to fully understand sugar in all its gooey glory, we need to have a little lesson in terminology to fully appreciate its pervasiveness.

In the 30,000-foot (9,145 m) bird's-eye view of nutrition, you have the macronutrients—fats, proteins, and carbohydrates. These are broken down in the body into the micronutrients—fatty acids (and glycerol), amino acids, and glucose, respectively. Sugar fits into the category of carbohydrates.

CARBOHYDRATES

Good carbs, bad carbs, no carbs, low carbs, high carbs, Atkins diet. I know you've heard of all these terms in relation to carbohydrates, but what is a carb, really? Simply put, it's the sugary (think birthday cakes and fruit) or starchy (spaghetti, bread, potato) part of foods. Sugars can be further classified as simple or complex carbohydrates.

SIMPLE CARBS

These are naturally occurring carbohydrates, like the lactose in milk and the fructose in fruit. But simple carbs also include human-manipulated sugars, the sugary bad carbs we all love to indulge in, like high-fructose corn syrup (and its many aliases) and sucrose. Also called "refined carbs," these simple carbs encompass white flour and everything that's made from it as well, plus white rice, which is rice stripped of its fiber. Simple carbs may have started as one of nature's whole foods, but no more. After we toyed with them—removing the fiber and destroying the minerals, vitamins, phytonutrients, and enzymes as we transformed them into white sugar, white flour, white rice, packaged cookies, baked goods, candies, sodas, fruit juices, snack foods, and even that blueberry muffin you have every morning with your coffee—they became a dangerous burden to our brains and our bodies. These fast-absorbing, fast-energy sugars

can cause a major spike in blood sugar, especially if consumed in high amounts, as most of us do in our society today.

COMPLEX CARBS

Unrefined, fiber-rich vegetables, legumes, and truly whole, unrefined grains (not stripped of their bran and germ) are called complex carbs. Because they are unrefined, these starches are full of vitamins, minerals, phytonutrients, enzymes, proteins, and other good stuff (unless you mess with them), and they take longer to digest. Thus, they do not cause a high spike in your blood sugar. Starch metabolism begins in your mouth, as the enzymes in your saliva convert these complex carbs into the sugar maltose. When maltose reaches the small intestine, it's converted into glucose. Since this is a longer process than the metabolism of simple carbs, complex carbs are considered time-release carbs; they don't offer that immediate spike in your blood sugar and give you long, sustained energy.

● From Food to Fuel

There are other types of and many other ways to describe carbs, but for the purposes of the Rainbow Juice Cleanse, let's look at the sugars glucose, fructose, and sucrose. Your tainted tongue may not be able to tell the difference between these sugars, but your body certainly can. They all give you the same amount of energy per gram, but are processed and used differently throughout the body.

GLUCOSE

The energy source you were intended to run on, glucose—a simple sugar—is also referred to as blood sugar. It's the only source of sugar your brain can use, and it is the preferred source of energy for your cells. As the body breaks down the carbs you consume into glucose, glucose builds up in the blood and is burned up and used immediately by the brain and the cells in your body. If it is not needed at that time, it is stored in muscle cells and the liver (as glycogen) for later use. All of this action is guided by insulin, a hormone released by the pancreas, which sits behind your stomach. Glucose also stimulates leptin, a hormone that helps to suppress your appetite. But just because you (over)ate it doesn't mean you can use it, and that's where having too much sugar—and thus too much circulating insulin—can cause problems like diabetes.

> Glucose is the only source of sugar that your brain can use.

FRUCTOSE

Found naturally in many fruits and vegetables, fructose is also added in massive amounts to various foods and beverages in the form of high-fructose corn syrup (HFCS). Keep in mind that almost all HFCS is genetically modified and appears under the guise of many other names. Sodas and many carbonated drinks, fruit juices, yogurts, frozen diet meals, energy drinks— almost all processed foods—are loaded with fructose. This sugar has become an anathema in nutrition circles. It is very different from glucose in its metabolic pathway, and it is not the preferred energy source for the brain or the muscles. Fructose, unlike glucose, is metabolized 100 percent in the liver, and it is considered more fat-loving and fat-producing than glucose. It does not cause insulin to be released (so it doesn't promote an increase in blood sugar) or stimulate leptin, the good hormone that regulates energy intake, energy expenditure, and satiety.

Fructose is broken down into free fatty acids (FFAs), very-low-density lipo-protein (VLDL, or bad cholesterol), and triglycerides, which are stored as, ugh, fat. This can cause fatty liver disease (the sugarholic type), as well as insulin resistance and metabolic syndrome. Fructose also prompts the production of nasty waste products, such as uric acid, raising your blood pressure and leading to gout, which often manifests first as big toe pain. More than any other type of sugar, fructose precipitates all types of chronic disease, as well as wrinkles and signs of aging. If you only ingested fructose from fruits and veggies, as our ancestors did, there wouldn't be such a problem, but that is simply not the case today. Our society consumes fructose in massive, previously unheard-of quantities. Fructose has become our main source of sugar and our number one source of calories. As Dr. Robert Lustig, professor of pediatrics in the Division of Endocrinology at the University of California, San Francisco, says, "Consuming fructose is essentially consuming fat." Enough said!

Note: About 80 percent of ethanol—the alcohol found in alcoholic beverages—is metabolized by the liver (just as fructose is), stimulating the same formation of fat-free fatty acids, VLDL (bad cholesterol), and triglycerides. So, alcoholic beverages are not part of the Rainbow Juice Cleanse!

SUCROSE

More commonly called "table sugar," sucrose is harvested from sugarcane and sugar beets, most of which today are genetically modified. Sucrose is a disaccharide (meaning its molecular structure comprises two sugars—the prefix *di* means "two"). This is in contrast to glucose and fructose, whose chemical structure is made up of just one sugar molecule (called monosaccharides—the prefix *mono* means "one"). When sucrose is consumed, it is further broken down into its component sugar units, glucose and fructose (that is, sucrose = glucose + fructose). The body uses glucose in its usual manner, as its preferred energy source, and the fructose, considered extra energy if it's not immediately needed, is poured into the fat-making process, which was stimulated by insulin in response to glucose.

● How Do Fruits and Veggies Fit In?

Fruits contain mainly sugar (simple carbs) and mostly in the form of fructose, and most veggies contain mainly starches (complex carbs) with a few exceptions, such as corn and most root veggies, which also contain higher amounts of fructose than glucose.

Is There Sugar in That?

Thanks to today's chemists, the sugar nomenclature has exploded into many unrecognizable yet seemingly innocuous names. Sugar in its various high-sweetness guises graces the ingredient lists of hundreds of thousands of commonly consumed food products and store-bought juices. You have to really make a conscientious (and educated) effort to stay away from it and not be fooled. Go grab something off the pantry shelf or out of the fridge and see if any of these sneaky names for sugar are on this list. Most of these aliases are provided courtesy of the movie *Fed Up:*

THE MANY ALIASES OF SUGAR

- Agave Nectar
- Barbados Sugar
- Barley Malt
- Beet Sugar
- Brown Rice Sugar
- Brown Sugar
- Buttered Syrup
- Cane Juice
- Cane Sugar
- Caramel
- Carob Syrup
- Castor Sugar
- Coconut Nectar
- Coconut Sugar
- Confectioners' Sugar
- Corn Sweeteners
- Corn Syrup
- Corn Syrup Solids
- Crystalline Fructose
- Date Sugar
- Diastatic Malt
- Diastase
- Dehydrated Cane Juice
- Demerara Sugar
- Dextran
- Dextrose
- Erythritol
- Ethyl Maltol
- Florida Crystals
- Fructose
- Fruit Juice
- Fruit Juice Concentrate
- Galactose
- Glucose
- Glucose Solids
- Golden Sugar
- Golden Syrup
- Grape Sugar
- High-Fructose Corn Syrup (HFCS)
- Honey
- Icing Sugar
- Lactose
- Malt Sugar
- Maltodextrin
- Maltose
- Mannitol
- Maple Syrup
- Molasses
- Muscovado
- Panocha
- Raw Sugar
- Refiner's Syrup
- Rice Syrup
- Sorbitol
- Sorghum Syrup
- Sucanat
- Sucrose
- Sugar (granulated, white)
- Turbinado Sugar
- Xylitol
- Yacon Syrup
- Yellow Sugar

THE SWEET SCIENCE OF ADDICTION

The addictive nature of sugar is no secret, for many of you experience it on a daily basis. You love it; you hate it; you crave it. You're depressed about it. You are going to rid yourself of it once and for all, but you have no willpower. You make it through the day without any. Then somehow you find yourself in line at the drive-through of a local fast-food joint with a supersized soda in your hand, and you don't know how it got there. You have lost all control! You are addicted!

Sugar, the ultimate frenemy and legal drug, hijacks your brain, specifically the reward centers of your brain. Your brain on sugar reacts just as if you'd taken a hit of cocaine.

It's as if you have become a (legal) drug addict. The actual substance of abuse may be different and the relapses and eventual consequences may not be as severe, but the feeling and the effect on the brain are exactly the same.

All because of sugar.

SUGAR AND HORMONES

There is much to say about sugar—fructose, in particular—and its effect on hormones, the body's messenger molecules. But I just want to make a few key points.

Fructose doesn't make you feel full.
Recall that when fructose is metabolized, it does not trigger the normal insulin and leptin responses, as glucose does. These are the hormones that tell the brain you have had enough to eat, so if they're not working, you don't feel full and you just keep on eating.

Fructose makes you gain fat weight.
Since your internal *stop* button is never triggered, you keep eating or drinking fructose-laced food and drinks. All the while your liver synthesizes that fructose into a fatty mess of free fatty acids, bad cholesterol, and triglycerides.

In addition, the whole insulin catastrophe causes the adrenal glands on your kidneys to produce more of the hormone cortisol, aka the stress hormone. Cortisol may bring on thyroid hormone issues, sleep issues, sex hormone issues (leading to infertility in both sexes and low testosterone in men), hair loss, and cancer. The list goes on and on.

All because of sugar.

SUGAR AND NUTRIENT DEPLETION

Just as most drugs (over-the-counter and prescription) deplete your body of nutrients, so does this legal drug—refined sugar. Like a thief in the night, sugar taps into your body's supply of B vitamins, such as B_6, B_{12}, and folic acid (B_9), and vitamins C and E, as well as a host of others, and strips them clean. It also leeches calcium and magnesium from your teeth and bones.

All because of sugar, the antivitamin.

SUGAR: FEEDING MODERN DISEASE

Our love affair with sugar is slowly killing us. We are fatter than ever—many of us morbidly obese;—our immune system is shot; our teeth are falling out; our skin is saggy and wrinkled; our blood sugar is through the roof; our bones are weak; our heart is failing; but, hey, cancer is thriving, and so are the Big Disease industries.

All because of sugar.

SUGAR AND OBESITY: POURING ON THE POUNDS

According to the Centers for Disease Control (CDC), more than one-third of American adults, or 78.6 million people, are obese. Almost 40 percent of these obese adults are in the forty- to fifty-nine-year-old age range, with Louisiana having the highest prevalence of any state at 34.7 percent (Louisiana is one of the top sugar-producing states, too). No state has less than 20 percent of obese adults.

Our number one source of calories contributing to this obesity epidemic is soft drinks (fructose). We are, as a populace, pouring on the pounds (and the associated diseases) with soft drinks, sweet teas, and fruit juices, and we are digging our own graves at the same time. And the liquid candy industries are moving in on us in ways you never dreamed possible. Dayton, Ohio; Ocean City, Maryland; and Miami Beach have all inked deals making Coke the official soft drink of their cities. Talk about a takeover! If these cities aren't on Gallup's Fattest Cities list already, they certainly will be very, very soon.

I'm not going to sugarcoat it. Soft drinks are something you really need to stop consuming, cold turkey, now. We just learned how they (and their fructose) are turned into fat. What better reason do you need? And if you allow your children to drink them, you need to get a handle on that as well.

Remember, our number one source of calories is soft drinks. According to the CDC, 70 percent of our obese youth already have at least one risk factor for cardiovascular disease and are more likely to have prediabetes, sleep apnea, low self-esteem, and psychological problems. We are killing our children and ourselves.

All because of sugar.

SUGAR AND THE IMMUNE SYSTEM

Few people realize that ingesting the high quantities of sugar that we do has an immediate effect on our immune system, our body's protective mechanism. With a blood sugar level at 120 (high, but very common today), the ability of our knight-in-shining-armor protector cells (aka white blood cells) to destroy bacteria and viruses may be reduced by well over 50 percent. Whoa! So, taking that into consideration, based on the 2014 National Diabetes Statistics Report of those with diabetes and prediabetes, including seniors, 115.1 million people in the United States possess an immune system that pretty much couldn't protect them from a pack of flies. Totally pathetic.

All because of sugar.

SUGAR AND TOOTH DECAY

Sugar is notorious for promoting tooth decay and causing cavities. You may even have a mouthful of fillings from your childhood years.

It might surprise you to know that fruit juices are not your friend, either, when it comes to your teeth. According to Marvin Pantangco, DDS, a holistic dentist and head of the Center for Natural Dentistry in Encinitas, California, "A key to preventing tooth decay is to avoid sugars and acids found in our foods and drinks. Fruit juices are even a major contributor because of their high sugar content."

Over time, the sugar-bacteria relationship in our mouth can lead to bleeding, inflamed gums, a condition called periodontal disease. In the worst cases of periodontal disease, the gum tissue actually begins to pull away from your teeth, and the bacteria go to work destroying the underlying bone

> Our number one source of calories is soft drinks.

that helps support your teeth. There is also a link between periodontal disease and a number of other chronic health issues, such as heart disease, diabetes, and rheumatoid arthritis—all inflammatory diseases.

All because of sugar.

SUGAR AND DIABETES

I'm sure everyone reading this knows someone, even many people, with diabetes. It might even be you. Diabetes has become a global epidemic. The American Diabetes Association's 2014 annual report states that 29.1 million Americans have diabetes; that's about 9.3 percent of the population. Prediabetes affects some 86 million (51 percent of them seniors).

What's going on here?!

I don't want to minimize the importance of obesity and excess body fat as some of the most significant contributors to diabetes, nor the fact that insulin works much less effectively with a diet consisting of fatty foods, but for our purposes here, we are going to talk the sugar side of the equation.

Brian Clement, PhD, NMD, LN, co-director of the amazing Hippocrates Health Institute in West Palm Beach, Florida, helps diabetics balance their bodies daily at the institute. He notes that not only may diabetes be one of the most devastating diseases of all time, but also children are now being diagnosed with it at younger ages each year. Says Dr. Clement, "Diabetes just starts to eat up the body because the body cannot handle the high amounts of sugar in the blood all the time without erosion of the cells of the body. These poor kids—ten to fifteen years old—are now dealing with type-2 diabetes, where just two and three generations ago, we used to see sixty years of bad living before a person had that disease. Now it takes ten or fifteen years." Shocking!

Despite the toll diabetes is taking on our population and despite the conventional wisdom about diabetes, diabetes is reversible and no one knows that better than Gabriel Cousens, MD, a homeopathic physician and the founder of the Tree of Life Rejuvenation Center in Patagonia, Arizona. He wrote a book called *There Is a Cure for Diabetes* and starred in the 2009 documentary *Simply Raw*, which followed six people through a thirty-day program in an attempt to reverse their diabetes without medication. Check out the movie and see what happens to these six subjects. It's astounding.

Keep in mind that diabetes is not just a disease about blood sugar. Serious long-term complications, including heart disease, kidney failure, blindness, stroke, infections, amputations, erectile dysfunction, depression, and dementia, are prevalent among diabetics long term.

All because of sugar.

SUGAR AND OSTEOPOROSIS

Osteoporosis was traditionally a disease we didn't see until later in life, but today we are setting our children up for this condition much sooner by allowing them to consume too much liquid candy and sugar overall. Sugar destroys bones, as it is highly acidifying. Studies have shown that consuming excessive quantities of sugar causes a large increase in urinary calcium excretion (pulled from the bones!), both in healthy subjects as well as those who are prone to kidney stones.

All because of sugar.

SUGAR AND CARDIO-VASCULAR DISEASE

There is also a link between sugar and cardiovascular disease, as well as all its inflammatory relatives, including stroke, high blood pressure, high cholesterol, and even erectile dysfunction. Yes, I'm sorry to have to report that last one.

Sugar makes your blood sticky and more likely to clot. As Harvard Medical School pointed out in February 2014 on their Harvard Health Blog, "Over the course of [a] 15-year study, participants who took in 25 percent or more of their daily calories as sugar were more than twice as likely to die from heart disease as those whose diets included less than 10 percent added sugar. Overall, the odds of dying from heart disease rose in tandem with the percentage of sugar in the diet and that was true regardless of a person's age, sex, physical activity level, and body mass index."

All because of sugar.

SUGAR AND CANCER

Sugar feeds cancer. Numerous studies show that cancer cells can readily metabolize fructose, sparking their growth. That should be enough to stop you in your tracks and make you drop your soda.

All because of sugar.

EVEN MORE CONDITIONS CONNECTED TO SUGAR CONSUMPTION

Science has proven that each of these maladies is fed by all forms of sugar:

- Acne, Rosacea, Psoriasis, Eczema
- ADD (Attention Deficit Disorder), Dyslexia, Brain Fog
- ALS (Lou Gehrig's Disease)
- Alzheimer's
- Asthma
- Bipolar Disorder
- Candida (fungal yeast infection)
- Chronic Fatigue Syndrome
- Coronary Heart Disease
- Crohn's Disease, Diverticulosis, Diverticulitis, Leaky Gut Syndrome
- Depression
- Erectile Dysfunction
- Fibromyalgia
- Gallstones
- HIV
- Hypertension (high blood pressure)
- Infertility, Impotence, Sterility
- Menopause, Andropause
- Metabolic Syndrome
- Multiple Sclerosis
- Nonalcoholic Fatty Liver Disease
- Nutrient Deficiencies
- Osteoarthritis
- Parkinson's Disease
- Schizophrenia
- Sleep Apnea
- Stroke

SUGAR, WRINKLES, AND AGING SKIN

If you thought sugar was only doing a number on your insides, wait until you hear what my expert, Linda Chaé, has to say about how sugar promotes aging skin and wrinkles. First, a little background.

Sugar and high-GI foods cause systemic inflammation in the body, which is a tremendous contributor to accelerated aging, as well as chronic disease. Inflammation, in turn, produces heat and triggers enzymes that break down skin collagen, specifically elastin. This breakdown in collagen causes wrinkles. Elastase is a harmful, proinflammatory enzyme that breaks down and literally eats away at elastin, a key structural protein vital for elasticity—that springiness and youthfulness of skin tone.

This process, called glycation, results in a cross-linking of collagen, making it stiff and inflexible, like a scar. These scars are called advanced glycation end products (AGEs) and show up not only on the skin, but also internally. There is a correlation between these accumulating toxic AGEs and many diseases, including chronic inflammatory diseases, like diabetes, heart disease, cancer, and autoimmune diseases. Research even suggests that fructose is upwards of ten times more proficient than glucose at creating AGEs.

Linda Chaé of Chaé Manufacturing, creator of skin and body products that "do no harm," gives a few of the greatest analogies I've ever heard on this topic: "It's like when you are baking cookies and the dough develops a harder texture than what it was before it was put in the oven. Or, if you leave a rubber band out in the sun, it becomes hard and brittle, causing breakage—this is what also happens to our collagen. These examples illuminate the heat and enzyme breakdown that happens to the skin when large amounts of sugar are consumed. Younger, healthier skin can be achieved by eliminating sugar and a high glycemic diet. Avoiding sugar is one of the single most important rules for looking and feeling younger."

Linda also points out, "Sugar feeds yeast and bacteria, which contribute to numerous skin conditions, including acne, eczema, psoriasis, and dermatitis."

So the bottom line: That nasty enzyme elastase can be stimulated by consuming sugar. By eliminating sugar, you reduce inflammation, and you reduce the amount and activity of elastase, preventing skin from aging and preventing the onset of wrinkles. Many medicinal plants, as well as many of the powerful phytonutrients, such as quercetin, found in the Rainbow Juice Cleanse, are thought to do just that! Let's start youthing!

ARTIFICIAL SWEETENERS

I'm sure it won't surprise you that I don't approve of or consume any artificial sweeteners. "If man made it, don't eat it," said good ol' Jack LaLanne. Artificial sweeteners are worse for you than fructose in many ways. They are also neurotoxins, meaning they are toxic to your nervous system— your brain, your spinal cord, and your nerves. The blue packets, the pink packets, the yellow packets—I stay far away from all of them. So should you.

STEVIA: MOTHER NATURE'S MIRACLE SWEETENER

Stevia, derived from *Stevia rebaudiana* (aka the sweetleaf plant), is a natural sweetener and the only one I recommend in the Rainbow Juice Cleanse, due to its negligible effect on blood glucose. Its glycoside extracts are about three hundred times as sweet as sugar, so it only takes a small amount to produce the same sweetness as sugar. Stevia has been used as a sweetener for centuries in many cultures, including Japan, where today it accounts for 40 percent of the Japanese sweetener market.

Dr. Clement notes, "The sugar and sugar substitute industries have spent millions worldwide on preventing stevia's entrance into the marketplace. They actually resorted to fabricating propaganda claiming this healthy plant caused diseases like cancer. Only recently has it gained acceptance as a sugar substitute in the United States, but in many countries stevia is still outlawed. If it were not for the giant soda companies, who began to utilize it as a no-calorie additive, it would have been outlawed in the United States as well."

Stevia comes in several forms—plant, powder, and liquid drops. Does it taste exactly like sugar? No, and don't expect it to. But as your taste buds balance out, you will come to love it. I especially love the real stevia leaves fresh off the plant, which is very easy to grow. Be cautious of store-bought brands that use stevia along with table sugar or other added ingredients. The fresh stevia leaf, taken directly from the plant, is always best!

For those who choose to purchase it from the store or online, Donna Gates spells out the conversions from sugar to stevia in her book *The Stevia Cookbook*.

SUGAR-TO-STEVIA CONVERSIONS

Sugar	Stevia Drops	Stevia Powder
1 cup (200 ml)	1 teaspoon (5 ml)	1 teaspoon (5 ml)
1 tablespoon (15 ml)	6–9 drops	¼ teaspoon (1.3 ml)
1 teaspoon (5 ml)	2–4 drops	A pinch to $1/16$ teaspoon (0.3 ml)

We've Come for the Fruit!

Wow! With all this information, it should be obvious that you need to eliminate sugar from your diet now, in all its devilish forms, especially during the Rainbow Juice Cleanse. And I hope you will continue this trend afterward as well! I feel the same way about fruit-only juices: Give them up. Remember that the primary sugar in fruit is fructose. I do not recommend drinking fruit juice, especially store-bought, pasteurized fruit juice, but even if you just made a glass yourself with your own juicer, I'm not a fan. From a healing perspective, and that's where I come from, it is not ideal. There are so many better and equally delicious options. We just learned how fructose acts in the body, so it shouldn't be hard to see what that tall glass of orange juice is doing to you.

Fruit and fruit juices seem to be the common go-to foods for someone transitioning to a healthier diet, most often because that person already has a sugar addiction and these are just healthier versions (as I've been told by clients) of the same thing. But as with the bad sugars, people also tend to overdo and overeat fruit and fruit juices and consume fewer greens, sprouts, vegetables, and other less fructose-containing healthy foods. (Note: Eating too many fats, as in nuts, is another trap many fall into when transitioning to healthier eating.) Why people aren't just craving their greens, I will never know, but you will once you overcome your sugar addiction. I know I did.

Fruit today is not the way it was back in the days of the Garden of Eden. Some of our fruit is much bigger, easier to eat, and much, much sweeter (that is, packed with fructose). Over the past two hundred years or so, we, as a society, have played Food God, turning once heavenly health-givers into too much of a sweet thing. We've been breeding certain fruits selectively. As a result, grapefruit and seedless (and sterile) watermelons and grapes fill our grocery stores and farmer's markets today. They are a far cry from their wild and crazy ancestors.

Dr. Clement tells me, "The hybridized fruit of today has, on average, thirty times more sugar than its ancestral forebears."

> "The hybridized fruit of today has, on average, thirty times more sugar than its ancestral forebears."

On top of what we've already learned about fructose, that should get you thinking.

Let me make it clear: I'm not banning fruit here. I eat fruit myself, and fruits are part of the Rainbow Juice Cleanse foods and the Rainbow Juice Cleanse recipes. What I am doing is creating the awareness that eating whole fruit, with its fiber and full nutritional and phytonutrient package, is entirely different than drinking a glass of condensed fruit juice or even adding a few pieces of fruit in your veggie juice. This is especially true for someone facing a health challenge (as most of us are today) and for those trying to lose weight.

From a healing and weight loss perspective, try to keep your total fruit consumption between 5 and 10 percent of your total daily calorie intake. The cleaner and healthier you become, the better your body can handle fruits and even fruit juice. But most of us could use the sugar break. Work on building your health through greens and sprouts, soaked and sprouted nuts and seeds, and phytonutrient-rich veggies and their juices. And consume your fruit whole: Don't juice it!

> Try to keep your total fruit consumption between 5 and 10 percent of your total daily calorie intake.

HOW TO SHOP THE RAINBOW

TIME TO GO SHOPPING—and who doesn't love that? Here are the Rainbow Juice Cleanse rules you should follow.

● Avoid Pasteurized Juices

You may be all pumped up and ready to "get your squeeze on" with the Rainbow Juice Cleanse, and that's terrific! But don't think running to your local grocery or convenience store and picking up a bottle of juice you find there is going to cut it. I'm sorry to inform you that it won't. Store-bought juices have many issues, the first of which is that they have been pasteurized.

Commercial juice manufacturers and grocery and convenience-store retailers can thank Louis Pasteur for inventing the commercial pasteurization process. It prevents slow spoilage that is caused by microbial growth and allows for a much longer shelf life and a much higher bottom line for those industries.

But *you* can't thank Mr. Pasteur, because this high-heat—almost sterilization—process does nothing for your health or even your bottom line.

Heating juice destroys its nutrients, particularly water-soluble, heat-sensitive nutrients like vitamin C and all the B vitamins like thiamine (B_1), riboflavin (B_2), niacin (B_3), pantothenic acid (B_5), pyridoxine (B_6), biotin (B_7), folic acid (B_9), and cobalamin (B_{12}), and these are nutrients we definitely want in our juice! Heat also destroys phytonutrients, such as polyphenolics/phenols, as well as all the enzymes found in nature's foods, essentially giving you a dead juice. Don't waste your money on pasteurized juices.

Don't waste your money on pasteurized juices.

● Shop Smart When Choosing Your Produce

The Environmental Working Group (EWG), a nonprofit, nonpartisan consumer advocacy group, always has loads of great consumer health information on its website, Ewg.org. I particularly like the organization's yearly analysis of which nonorganic produce is the most laden with pesticides and which is the least.

In 2014, in single samples, EWG researchers found that grapes contained fifteen different pesticides, and cherry tomatoes, celery, and imported snap peas contained thirteen!

According to the EWG, the Environmental Protection Agency (EPA) has not complied in full with the congressional mandate to "assess pesticides in light of their particular dangers to children and to ensure that pesticides posed a reasonable certainty of no harm to children or any other high risk group." Nor has the EPA complied with the Consumer Right to Know Act, which requires the EPA to publish and distribute consumer information about this in grocery stores (the EPA stopped doing this in 2007). So, for the past decade, the EWG has published this information for consumers in its "Shopper's Guide to Pesticides in Produce." Here are the EWG's latest rankings.

THE DIRTY DOZEN

Buy these organic. They are the most pesticide-laden produce tested in 2014.

Apples	Cucumbers	Peaches	Spinach
Celery	Grapes	Potatoes	Strawberries
Cherry Tomatoes	Nectarines (imported)	Snap Peas (imported)	Sweet Bell Peppers

THE CLEAN FIFTEEN

Try to buy these organic, but you could get away with not buying these organic in a pinch. No single fruit sample from this list tested positive for more than four kinds of pesticides, which still makes me want to buy them organic or grow my own!

Asparagus	Cauliflower	Mangoes	Sweet Corn
Avocados	Eggplant	Onions	Sweet Peas, frozen
Cabbage	Grapefruit	Papayas	
Cantaloupe	Kiwi	Pineapple	Sweet Potatoes

Juice Fresh, Organic Produce

The Rainbow Juice Cleanse juices do not require any processing in your body; they are absorbed into your bloodstream very quickly. So it is important to use pesticide-, fungicide-, and herbicide-free produce—that means organic. In addition, it has been found that organic produce contains more nutrients than conventional, chemically "sprayed" produce. I only recommend juicing with organic produce.

Decipher the PLU Sticker

You know that little sticker you find on the produce you buy? That's called the PLU sticker, and you need to become an expert at interpreting it. The numbers on the PLU, or the "price look-up" sticker, reveal the most important thing you need to know about your precious food—how it was grown. Was it organically grown, sprayed with toxic chemicals, or genetically modified? See the PLU code rules below.

For example, the sticker on the banana I just bought reads 94011; this means it is organic. If it was sprayed with chemicals, the sticker would say 4011, and if it was genetically modified (and most likely also sprayed with chemicals), the sticker would read 84011.

Armed with this information, you are one step closer to good health.

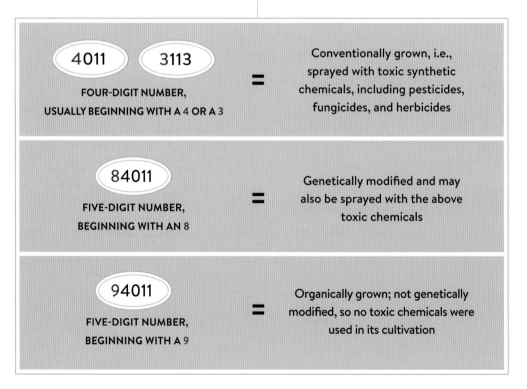

4011 3113	=	Conventionally grown, i.e., sprayed with toxic synthetic chemicals, including pesticides, fungicides, and herbicides
FOUR-DIGIT NUMBER, USUALLY BEGINNING WITH A 4 OR A 3		
84011	=	Genetically modified and may also be sprayed with the above toxic chemicals
FIVE-DIGIT NUMBER, BEGINNING WITH AN 8		
94011	=	Organically grown; not genetically modified, so no toxic chemicals were used in its cultivation
FIVE-DIGIT NUMBER, BEGINNING WITH A 9		

Watch Your Grocery Costs Plummet

One of the complaints I hear when I talk to people about eating healthy is that they cannot afford it. I get where they are coming from. Fast-food (or fat food) is cheap. But what you need to understand—and, I assure you, Big Food understands it—is this: Unhealthy food is nutritionally void, leaving you constantly hungry, constantly eating, and constantly purchasing more food. Healthy food, on the other hand, is so nutrient-dense it leaves your body and cells satisfied, so you are not hungry and you purchase less food.

Change Up Your Produce Often

The whole idea behind juicing is to load your body up with a variety of fresh, organic, alkaline nutrients, so constantly change the types of veggies you juice to give your body the full spectrum of nutrients. Be sure to choose seasonal and local produce as much as possible.

Unfamiliar Ingredients

In this book, there are a handful of ingredients that may be new to you, but are essential in your health journey and are a part of the Rainbow program. Ingredients such as Nama Shoyu, carob powder, nutritional yeast, AFA, and sea veggies such as dulse and kelp can all be purchased at your local health food store and/or online, as can any other unfamiliar ingredient.

HOW TO SHOP FOR A JUICER

When buying a juicer, there are two schools of thought:

1 *Buy a great-quality juicer that costs a little more, but will last a lifetime.*

2 *Buy a lower-priced juicer, because if it's anything like my treadmill, chances are I won't stick with it.*

I'm here to motivate you to stick with it and to make juicing part of your normal, daily routine, even after the cleanse. But I do understand your desire to buy an affordable juicer in the beginning, so as not to make this new venture too costly.

There isn't any one "right" juicer when you start out. I just want you to buy one you will use! Juicers can range in price from $50 for a low-end model to $2,000 for a commercial-grade juicer found at juice bars, but any juicer can get you started. Choose one that fits your budget and lifestyle. Just realize that over time the motor in an inexpensive juicer will most likely burn out, and you will have to buy another one. In addition, with the very low-priced models, you may have to re-juice the pulp several times to get all the juice out of the fiber. Perhaps the second time around, when you become a veteran "juicer," you will be ready to invest in a better-quality juicer for your juicing future.

TYPES OF JUICERS
Here are the various types of juicers on the market:

• **CENTRIFUGAL JUICER:** This popular style of juicer is found in many department and discount stores. It works at high speeds, pushing produce through its shredder disc, grating it, and then expelling the pulp through a strainer basket and squeezing out the juice—much like your washing machine spin cycle. This juicer will not juice wheatgrass, and you must roll leafy greens into a ball and push them through for juicing. This type of juicer tends to have the fastest cleanup, is usually less expensive, and runs at higher RPMs (revolutions per minute), producing juice fast.

• **MASTICATOR JUICER:** This juicer grates the produce, then masticates it (chews up the pulp), and finally squeezes out the juice. This type of juicer can also make sauces and nut butters with the blank-plate attachment that's included with the juicer. It runs at lower RPMs, which is said to lessen the oxidation of the juice, producing a higher-quality juice.

• **HYDRAULIC PRESS JUICER:** This type of juicer slowly presses the juice out of produce and introduces the least amount of oxygen into the juice. Thus, it is said to produce the least amount of oxidation and a very high-nutrient juice.

• **WHEATGRASS JUICER:** This is specifically for making wheatgrass juice and comes in electric and manual models. This is not for juicing fruits or veggies. Some of the masticator juicers and presses will also juice wheatgrass.

• **CITRUS JUICER:** This type of juicer is exclusively for juicing citrus fruits, such as oranges and grapefruit, and is not used in this book's juicing recipes. However, it can be used in some of the food recipes (see chapters 10 to 13). Alternatively, you can juice citrus fruits by hand.

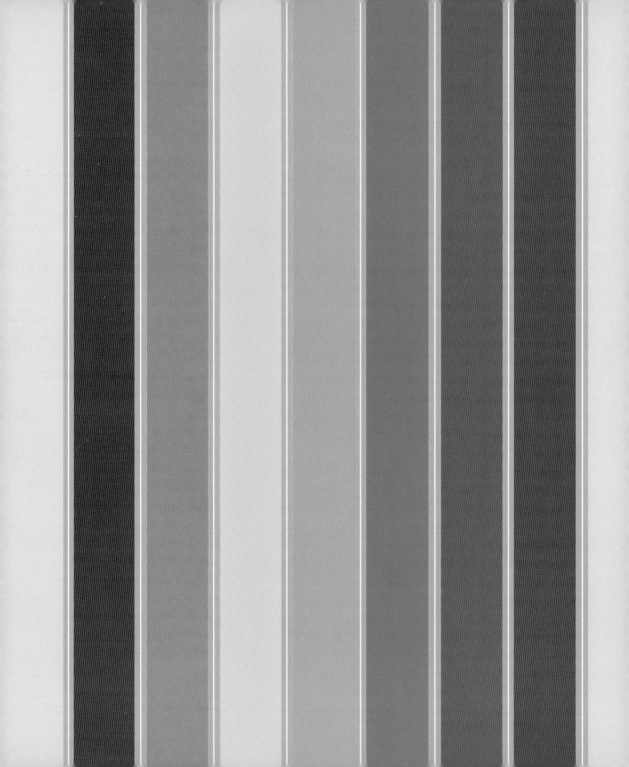

4

THE RAIN BEFORE THE RAINBOW

YOUR BODY IS CONTINUOUSLY PRODUCING TOXINS and metabolic wastes on a daily basis, and your natural detoxification systems can handle this when you eat nature's diet of mostly raw, organic, alkaline foods. If you've been riding a bit too long on the highly toxic Standard American Diet (SAD) train, though, you may encounter a few bumpy patches and layovers along the way to your final destination: the Rainbow. Remember what Dolly Parton says: "If you want the rainbow, you've got to put up with the rain."

American Diet Disasters

Americans have, let's just say, a puzzling love affair with food. The Standard American Diet (SAD) is characterized by its gluttonous excesses of sugar—particularly fructose—and other refined carbohydrates, trans and saturated fats, mucus-forming dairy, massive amounts of processed meats, acrylamides, aspartame, and MSG, with a piece of pesticide-laden iceberg lettuce and a slice of genetically modified tomato on top. This is certainly a lesson in the value of quantity over quality. Yes, a pretty sad state for the Standard American Diet.

But don't forget its creative spin-off for the real explorers of food—the State Fair Diet. In this eating regimen, fairgoers choose from tempting "delicacies" like Kool-Aid Pickles, Pop Rocks Doughnuts, Pickle Pops, Beer Gelato, Hot Beef Sundaes, Krispy Kreme Burgers, Beer-Battered Bacon, any kind of food you can imagine on a skewer like Porkabello Kabobs or even Elvis on a Stick. And don't forget the merciless deep-fried everything, including Deep-Fried Twinkies, Deep-Fried Pineapples, Deep-Fried Bacon-Wrapped Turkey Leg, and Deep-Fried Bubble Gum, for which fairgoers spend a fortune.

Just reading those lists is enough to make me have a reversal of my own fortune. You would think we would be nutritionally thriving, living in the land of the plenty, but that's just not the case. The danger of being stuffed has been realized, but so has the danger of being starved.

Deanna Latson, MA, CCN, nutritionist, founder, and chief product officer at Ariix, a company with innovative and leading-edge health and wellness prod-ucts, points out, "You don't have to live in a developing country to be starving. We as a nation are overfed and certainly overweight and obese, but we are woefully malnourished. The foods most people subsist on comprise an unnatural diet and empty calories that actually deplete our body's vital nutrients and leave us constantly walking around hungry."

Many of our fad diets have the same effect. Whenever my good friend Woodson Gardner was on a diet—and she's tried them all, from the Thin Mints Diet to the Dude, Where's My Gut? Diet, even the Let's Lose the Caboose Diet (I know, where does she find these?!)—she would always say to me, "Stay back, girlfriend, I'm on a new diet this week and I'm hangry!" What she meant was she was hungry and angry! I could tell this was not a good combination at all. Her diets were tasteless, super-restrictive, and provided no real nourishment whatsoever (Thin Mints?). She couldn't stop cheating because she was always hungry. Or hangry, rather. Not a fun way to live.

> We as a nation are overfed, overweight, and woefully malnourished.

So when you finally decide you've had enough of the Jelly-Belly roller coaster and you want to try the Quit Eating the Crappy Foods Diet or, better yet, the Rainbow Juice Cleanse, you'll need to jump over a few small hurdles on your way to reaching the treasures at the end of the rainbow.

The Healing Crisis Explained

On the road to becoming healthier and reaching the pot of gold at the end of the rainbow, it is not uncommon for people to experience what is called a "healing crisis" (also called Herxheimer Reaction), a natural and normal process of "spring cleaning," so to speak, that your toxic body may experience when you give it a rest from the SAD and begin your healthy eating and juicing journey. When you stop shoveling in heavily processed, pesticide-laden foods and drinks, and you give your cells a breather, they can finally celebrate and begin to unload their wastes into circulation for final elimination. In addition, a massive die-off and purge of pathogenic organisms (Candida yeast, viruses, bad bacteria) may occur. Sometimes, however, the debris expulsion is so fast that the organs of elimination—the skin,

liver, bladder, kidneys, lungs, sinuses, and GI tract—cannot keep pace. During this period, every system in the body is working to eliminate toxins and set up for healthy regeneration, so you may experience some cleansing symptoms for a few days.

Keep in mind, the longer the toxins and pathogens stay in your body, the worse your overall health, and the faster you develop disease and gain weight. You have set up the perfect internal environmental storm for disease to thrive and your fat cells to distend so you cannot lose weight. And then, of course, you won't fit into that Herve Leger bandage dress.

COMMON DETOX SYMPTOMS

The healing crisis symptoms are unique to each individual and all over the map—some mild, some more severe—and some lucky ducks experience none at all.

Here's the good, the bad, and the ugly:

The Ugly: Worst news first, and this may never happen to many of you, but since your body uses every outlet available to get clean, I need to mention the possibilities. You may feel nauseated. Ugh, not the best feeling in the world, but this can happen when you eliminate sugar, caffeine, and other toxins, as they look for their proper exit signs. You may experience a little more frequent bowel activity. OK, that was a nice way of saying possible diarrhea, but if the Big Pipe hasn't been cleaned in a while, the broom (fibrous fruits and veggies) is surely going to sweep it clean. This is not a bad thing. Stagnant eliminations get reabsorbed back into the bloodstream. Get 'em out!

You may see skin eruptions. No, this is not the most glamorous part of the healing crisis, but pimples or redness is something you may experience as you eliminate harmful substances from your diet, especially dairy and gluten. It might surprise you to know that high and low emotions may also get stirred up and flushed outward. Your loved ones might find you just a little bit grumpy. If you experience any of these reactions, alert your household members to come out from their hiding places, because the symptoms should diminish after a few days.

Once your blood sugar stabilizes and your body goes through its first round of housecleaning, all these symptoms should subside.

The Bad: You may experience a runny nose as toxins use every available escape route. Let it flow; get it out! Use a neti pot, if you must! You may feel fatigue and low energy, especially if you're eliminating sugar from your diet; your body is using all its available mojo to rid itself of rubbish. You may have mild headaches, particularly if you are eliminating caffeine (which is highly recommended), as your blood vessels are rebounding back to their normal and healthy circumference, having been forever dilated from the multiple daily cups of Joe or soda caffeine IV drips.

The Good: You're bursting with energy! You have a strong sense of emotional freedom: You feel clearer, more alert, and in control! You feel cleaner inside and out. You are supercharged and ready to kick-start life! You may not start in this phase, but you certainly should end up here after the cleanse, so everyone should look forward to this.

HELP FOR THE HEALING CRISIS

The Herxheimer Reaction is usually just a bump in the road and resolves itself within a few days. In rare cases, however, if these symptoms are too much to bear, you may need to see your doctor. You may have a previously unknown underlying issue that is rearing its ugly head and needs to be addressed. Most of you, however, will want to slow down the symptoms just a bit or help further facilitate your body's own natural cleansing systems. There are many steps you can take to do so that will still keep you on track to the rainbow's pot of gold. Many of these steps are utilized by renowned healing centers and spas.

A little downtime, if you can spare it, will help expedite the cleansing and detoxification process.

Get some extra rest. A little downtime, if you can spare it, will help expedite the cleansing and detoxification process. Sleep in a little longer than usual on Saturday and Sunday mornings; go to bed earlier each night; or take a quick catnap during the day, if your schedule permits. Put a few drops of lavender oil on your hands and rub them on your pillow or an eye mask and let the aroma soothe you into a deep slumber as your body goes to work for you.

Start dry skin brushing. Your skin plays a huge role in daily detoxification and receives a third of all the blood that circulates throughout your body. So help it along with a natural bristle brush. You'll shed dry skin cells, improve vascular and lymphatic circulation, and stimulate nerve endings. This will get the impurities moving along.

Get chiropractic adjustments and acupuncture treatments. Utilizing the body's innate intelligence, both of these modalities help align and restore the body's nerve signals and/or energy pathways, bringing your body back in balance. We are vibrations of energy, yet most of us ignore or forget to take care of this vital aspect of our being, which can aid in cleansing and balancing the body as a whole.

Indulge in a massage. Now here's your excuse to get a massage, and it's a good one: Think of your muscles, tissues, and organs as sponges holding stagnant wastes. A massage squeezes out those sponges and gets those nasty wastes moving and flowing into the circulatory system for a major exodus. Keep calm and go book a massage! Massage day is my favorite day of the week.

Utilize aromatherapy and essential oils. According to the National Association of Holistic Aromatherapy, aromatherapy is "the art and science of utilizing naturally extracted aromatic essences from plants to balance, harmonize, and promote the health of the body, mind, and spirit." And who doesn't need all of that during a cleanse? Pick out a scent that appeals to you, or try some of the more well-known calming and detoxifying aromas, like lavender, eucalyptus, or bergamot fruit oil. Place a few drops, mixed in a base oil, on the back of your neck or temples, through your hair, on your pillow, on the bottom of your feet, in a warm bath, or use it as a body lotion—the uses are endless!

Zen out in hot yoga classes. This is one of my favorite past times. You get a killer workout, a big-time sweat detox, stimulation and cleansing of every internal organ, and your mind snags a serene meditative state—all in one hour. I feel like a new woman in an invincible state of bliss when I leave my daily hot yoga class. Give it a try!

Tranquilize in hot epsom salt baths. Epsom salt contains magnesium sulfate, a known detoxifier that will also help ease stress and muscle aches.

Unwind in infrared sauna sessions. Some of the best things in life make you sweat, and this is one of those things. Unlike traditional saunas, infrared saunas heat *you*, not the air, and it is a totally breathable and bearable heat. The infrared waves penetrate several inches deep into your muscles, increasing the circulation and getting oxygen into tissues and toxins out. Make sure it is also a low-EMF (electromagnetic frequency) sauna. I spend at least thirty minutes in mine, three to five times a week—sometimes more.

Simmer in steam baths. Detoxification of our water-based organs—lungs, kidneys, and bladder—takes place in a steam bath. Utilize geranium rose flower oil or other aromatherapy essential oils while you steam as well.

Luxuriate in whirlpool baths. The whirlpool action puts significant pressure on the lymphatic system, a major part of your immune system, which has no pump to move itself. You have lymph vessels and lymph nodes all over your body that suck metabolic wastes from the extracellular spaces, but the lymph can get congested and stagnant if it doesn't move. Whirlpool baths promote that circulation. Be sure chlorine or other harmful chemicals aren't used in the bath. Ozone would be one of the best options.

Jump on a rebounder. This is another excellent mover and shaker of the lymphatic system. Just a twenty-minute session on this personal mini-trampoline should be enough to get your detox machine moving, as you work against consistent gravitational pressure while bouncing.

Perform some kind of exercise. Any time you sweat, including while engaging in mild exercise, you increase your body's circulation. This prompts your skin, colon, and lymphatic system to release toxins. Those new to cleansing, however, may not be able to maintain their normal energetic pace during the seven-day Rainbow Juice Cleanse, so the decision about whether or not to exercise during this phase should be based on your energy levels and how you feel. Avoid strenuous exercise for sure, and stay well-hydrated. You should, however, be able to go for a brisk walk, jump on the rebounder, or even do some stretching or take a yoga class—at your own pace. But if you feel you must rest during the seven days because you are feeling the effects of the healing crisis, reserve your energy and resume your exercise regimen after the cleanse, when you are bouncing out of bed and feeling up to the task.

Take a colonic. Yes, I know this is a touchy subject for some, and it is certainly not required. But if you're one of those brave souls who do choose to engage in colon hydrotherapy during the seven-day Rainbow Juice Cleanse, you will notice a difference. Healthy bacteria cannot colonize in a toxic colon, so the removal of long-standing, blocked, toxic waste matter from the colon will allow the good bacteria to recolonize and flourish. After a colonic, your large intestine is better equipped to assimilate nutrients and eliminate toxic wastes quickly and efficiently. Many experience increased energy after a colonic— I know I do.

> While cleansing, avoid strenuous exercise for sure, and stay well-hydrated.

Get some sun. Exposing our skin to direct sunlight allows it to make that vital nutrient vitamin D, which boosts our immune system and protects us against various cancers. It's also a great way to commune with nature. Try to get at least fifteen to thirty minutes of sunshine a day; the best way to get vitamin D into your body is on skin without sunscreen. This should give you enough radiation to produce about 10,000 international units of the vitamin. (If you are concerned about sunburn or have any medical concerns, avoid the peak UV periods of the day between 10 a.m. and 3 p.m. For times when you spend more than thirty minutes in the sun, Ewg.org has a great list of non-toxic sunscreens you may want to try.)

Drink more clean water. Make sure the water you drink is nonchlorinated, nonfluoridated, filtered water. (I use a water filter with a zeolite wall that attracts bacteria, viruses, parasites, and protozoa and kills them and also destroys heavy metals, chlorine, fluoride, pharmaceuticals, and other toxins. See FatFuneralDetox.com for more information.) Keep the clean water flowing to help carry off toxins. Infuse it with lemons to further increase the elimination effects and get things moving. Carry that filtered lemon water with you everywhere in a BPA-free and phthalate-free bottle (plastic toxins that can seep into the water and your body) and keep flushing!

Eat mildly cooked, healthy foods. Cooked food slows down cleansing, and raw food speeds it up. If you are feeling some of the healing crisis symptoms and want to slow down the cleansing effects, eat some steamed broccoli or some sprouted bread with almond butter to slow down the healing crisis until you feel you can get back on the cleansing train again.

Consume juice-boosting extras. Certain supplements and foods are known to help minimize detox symptoms as well as facilitate cleansing. Many of these can be added to your Rainbow juices or included in the foods you eat. I've divided them into two categories: juice-boosting supplements and juice-boosting foods.

> Cooked food slows down cleansing, and raw food speeds it up.

JUICE-BOOSTING SUPPLEMENTS

Here are some of the things I look for in good cleansing supplements, all of which can enhance your progress in the Rainbow Juice Cleanse. Add them to your juice or consume separately.

• **ENZYMES:** Found naturally in unprocessed raw fruits, veggies, nuts, seeds, and sprouts, enzymes have many roles in the body. More than three thousand enzymes have been identified. Your pancreas also produces enzymes. Some (called proteolytic enzymes) gobble up debris intracellularly; others (known as digestive enzymes) microchomp your food into highly absorbable chunks extracellularly to aid in digestion. You can also find these enzymes in supplement form. Many people consume them on a daily basis, particularly during a cleanse.

• **HOMEOPATHIC FORMULAS:** Over two hundred years old, homeopathic remedies aid and stimulate the body's defense and immune responses, and reinforce the body's own natural healing capacity. You can find some great homeopathic weight-loss formulations

on the market—and note, these are hormone-free. Some that I've worked with significantly control hunger pangs and overeating, especially during the first few days of the cleanse or during the Rainbow Warm-Up and the Rainbow Rev-Up.

• **PEA PROTEIN, CRANBERRY PROTEIN, or ALMOND PROTEIN POWDER:** These easily digestible powders are high in plant-based proteins and colon-cleansing fiber. In my plant-powered protein powders, I like to incorporate a blend of probiotics (good bacteria that aid in bad pathogen die-off), prebiotics (food for probiotics), and enzymes (to aid in digestion). Look for dairy-free, soy-free, gluten-free, low-glycemic, and genetically modified organism (GMO)-free versions with no artificial colors or flavors, and make sure the product has been heavy metal–tested (free from mercury, lead, arsenic, and other health-poisoning metals contaminating our food, water, air, and many commercial products).

- **PSYLLIUM HUSKS:** The outer hull of the seeds of the *Plantago ovata* plant, psyllium husks are a soluble fiber that acts like a big broom in your intestines. Be sure to load up on the clean, filtered water when you're consuming psyllium husks. You can add a scoop to your juice. Psyllium husks absorb water and expand in the intestines, so this supplement scrubs down the intestinal tract as it makes things move out freely. Be sure to use only a small amount (about a tablespoon) and load up on water throughout the day to keep it moving through.

- **SPIRULINA, CHLORELLA, AND AFA (APHANIZOMENON FLOS-AQUAE) FRESHWATER ALGAES:** These superfood algaes are incredibly nutrient-dense. They have more protein per serving than any other organism (plant or animal) and provide tremendous nutrition in its simplest form. They help to balance blood sugar, aid in oxygen processing, extract heavy metals, and cleanse and detox the liver, bowel, and bloodstream.

- **ZEOLITE:** Used for hundreds of years throughout Asia, zeolite, a volcanic mineral, has a negatively charged honeycomb structure, which literally traps positively charged harmful elements—such as heavy metals, radioactive chemicals, and even lactic acid from sore, overworked muscles—and eliminates them from the body. Be sure to look for micronized (therapeutic quality), not milled (commercial grade) zeolite.

JUICE-BOOSTING FOODS

The list of cleansing foods found in nature is extensive, but here are a few you can add to the juice recipes (and foods) in this book if they are not already called for in the recipe.

- **CAYENNE PEPPER:** Composed of pure hot chiles, cayenne pepper peps up your circulation (you may sweat!) and your digestive system. It can also break up congestion. But did you know it is a superb remedy for headaches, too? Remember that a little pinch of cayenne pepper goes a long way, so take it one pinch at a time.

- **CHIA SEEDS:** The ancient superfood of the Aztecs and Mayans, chia seed has a mucilaginous fiber that helps to regulate the digestive system, as well as to stabilize blood sugar levels. High in plant-based and heart-healthy omega-3 fatty acids, as well as easily absorbable calcium and magnesium, chia seeds need to be soaked or sprouted (see next page) to harness their full value.

- **CILANTRO:** One of the most detoxifying green herbs, this immune-enhancing, cancer-fighting plant can expel heavy metals from the body, aid in digestion, and balance blood sugar. Keep in mind, however: It is mildly laxative.

- **GARLIC:** This natural antibiotic helps to normalize blood pressure and keep your blood clean! It's antibacterial and antifungal and also helps oust heavy metals from their hiding places in the body. Although the taste is sharp, fresh is always best, for it loses its potency dramatically, even when it's bottled in water or oil, or roasted or cooked.

- **GINGERROOT:** Who among us doesn't like a little ginger in our life? Add some of this pungent root to your juice to help alleviate nausea and expedite movement through the digestive tract. But keep in mind that it's a potent anti-inflammatory, with properties similar to NSAIDs (non-steroidal anti-inflammatory drugs). It also adds great flavor! And you can leave the peel on if you'd like.

- **OREGANO:** This herb's oils inhibit the growth of bacteria and Candida, and help clear mucus from the respiratory system, so it's great for that runny nose you may be experiencing during your healing crisis. Use it in your juices and on your food, and even put a few drops of oregano oil on your toothbrush for a fresh, clean, bacteria-free mouth.

- **SEA VEGETABLES:** These veggies are high in protein and easily absorbable, plus they're alkaline, and filled with bone-building trace minerals. Add a teaspoon of dulse, kelp, alaria, laver, nori powder, or any other veggie of the sea in place of salt or as a great flavor enhancer. Powerful sources of iodine and chlorophyll, sea veggies have a mucilaginous fiber that stabilizes blood sugar and hauls heavy metals from the body.

- **SPROUTS:** Sprouting releases loads of nutrients that would normally stay dormant in the seed, creating an incredible, living superfood! Anytime a seed is about to grow into a plant, it has the most nutrition it will ever have in that one little inch-long (2.5 cm) sprout. Take advantage of that, and use sprouts everywhere! I'm not talkin' boring alfalfa sprouts, either. I'm talkin' sunflower sprouts, broccoli sprouts, pea sprouts, cabbage sprouts, radish sprouts, wheatgrass sprouts—the list goes on and on. Do a little research, and get those sprouts in your juice and in your daily diet.

Here's how to sprout: Put the nuts/seeds/legumes in a mason jar, fill it with filtered water, and put on an airtight lid. Let it sit overnight or for a few hours so the water can soak in. Strain the water off (you can use a mason jar sprouting lid for this) and fill the jar with filtered water once again to rinse your nuts/seeds/legumes. Then discard the water. Put the jar top-side down and place it in the refrigerator in a bowl or tray or something that can catch any dripping, excess water. Rinse and drain the nuts/seeds/legumes every six hours or so (this timing doesn't have to be exact—just rinse them twice a day) for one to four days, or until you see the sprouts start to pop. Store them in the fridge and enjoy them on salads, in juices, or as added super-nutrients in any of your meals.

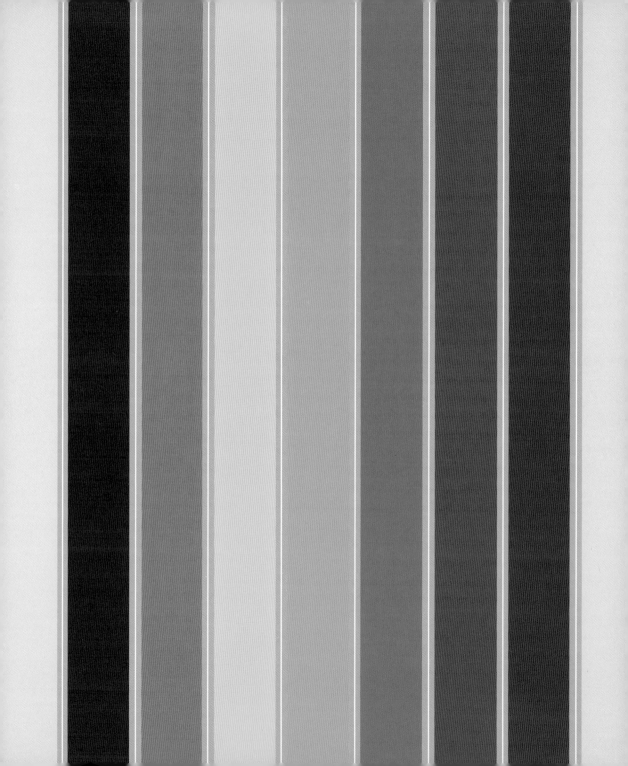

5

THE TREASURE AT THE END OF THE RAINBOW

ONCE YOU HAVE INFUSED YOUR BODY with lush foods and liquid sunshine juices, scraped the sludge from your pipes, and developed a new attitude and mind-set—game on! Your pot of gold awaits you! Wonderful things are happening!

This is what you have to look forward to. Read it now so you know what to expect. Use it as motivation throughout the Rainbow Juice Cleanse, but be sure to come back to it after the cleanse, read it again, and see how many apply to you! You may even have some new treasures of your own to add.

Let's open that treasure chest now.

Weight Loss and Inches Lost

OMG! You just tried on that dress, that shirt, or those skinny jeans, and now they fit! Just one week ago you looked like a stuffed sausage in them, and now you can at least feel good wearing them in public. If you continue eating the Rainbow Juice Cleanse foods and following the Rainbow recipes, along with drinking a Rainbow juice on a daily basis, those clothing items might actually become too big! Imagine that! It's certainly possible—it happened to me!

No more diets; no more counting calories. This is your new way of life.

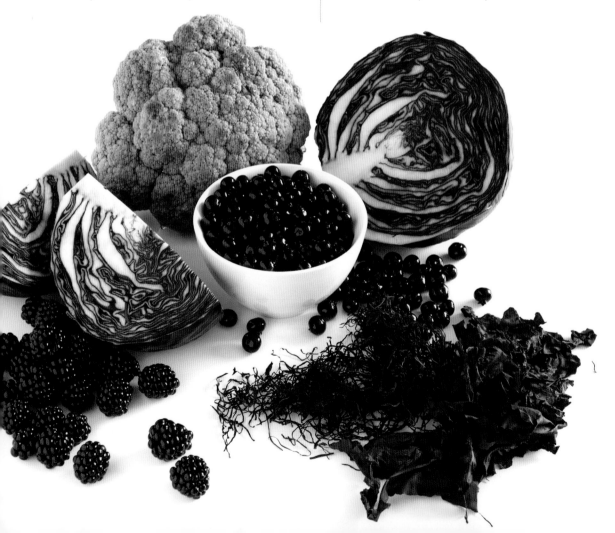

Your system is clean; you've jumped on the weight loss train; and that train is moving at full speed ahead! If you eat the way you've always eaten, you will have the body you have always had—there's no way around it! So end the vicious cycle now.

Taste Bud Transformation

Your taste buds have reset! Having been off processed foods for at least a week now, you will notice, if you slip back into an old food or drink habit, the foods and drinks you previously relished just don't taste right anymore. Don't go back! This is your inner voice (and your taste buds) screaming, "No more!" Don't slither back to the dark side. You have given your body the chance to finally appreciate real, clean, natural food, and it's thanking you!

Blood Sugar Balancing

There is no doubt that your blood sugar has stabilized. This program delivers a solid right hook to the sugar demons. If you are following the program, your blood sugar should become stable within just a few days. It's liberating not to feel those manic highs and terrible lows throughout the day, and not to be running to find your next sugar fix for a quick pick-me-up.

Increased Energy and Improved Men's Stamina

You are bouncing off the walls with energy! You are crushing it in your workouts! You feel exhilarated and liberated, and you are totally addicted to this new path to abundant health. You want to learn more about this way of living and plan to immediately cut down on your consumption of bad foods you may still be hanging on to (coffee; that chocolate bar you pick up while you're in line at the grocery store; the bag of chips you eat while watching *The Biggest Loser*). If you're a man, you may also have noticed improved stamina in the bedroom. Hmm, think about it: Erectile dysfunction is nothing but heart disease in another location (you know where), so if you have a detoxed body and clean blood, it can flow everywhere! And women, if you like the sound of that, get your man on the program with you now!

Dramatically Improved Skin

I love this one. When you consume Rainbow foods and juices, your skin will totally glow! Your skin cells turn over pretty fast, so if you give your body nourishing food, the next batch of skin cells you make will be nourished, glowing, and as soft as a baby's bottom. If you experienced some skin eruptions during the cleanse, remember that this is your body pushing out impurities and toxins by every means possible. Keep the toxins flowing, and there will soon come a day when people stop you on the street and ask you, "What do you use on your skin? It's glowing!" It happens to me all the time.

Overall Body Balancing

When you feed your body the proper foods and it finally gets nourishment at a cellular level, as you do in the Rainbow Juice Cleanse, your body's systems become balanced and operate optimally. I've seen it happen over and over again. You may notice that various symptoms you had in the past are no longer apparent or are starting to dissipate fast. Chronic issues resolve. If you are taking any kind of medication, do

not stop taking it on your own. Be sure to work with your doctor, as there are many medications that have to be tapered down slowly. If your health begins to improve and you see great results on your bloodwork (as I expect), your doctor should be very happy and willing to work with you on getting you off your meds.

Emotional Stabilization and Mental Clarity

Once you get off the sugar roller coaster and have stable blood sugar, a sense of emotional balance and mental focus takes over. Keep in mind, it took years to toxify your body, so it may take some time to work through the deeper layers of muck. It's like peeling an onion, and, thanks to you, the first layer is now long gone. The next layer may push out more than just old Doritos and birthday cake; it may push out some unexpected emotions as well. For many, this cleanse can be an emotional journey and transformation. This is common when the body undergoes a cleanse. Those emotions you stuffed away with that chocolate milk shake, supersized fries, and apple pie on the way to pick up your kids from school now desperately need an escape route so you can feel at peace again and in line with your new lifestyle. Go for a run, do some hot yoga, take a CrossFit class, or just cry it out. Let those old emotions go and make way for happy!

Improved Spirituality and Deeper Connections

Raw, unprocessed foods and juices have an energy, a vibration, and an aura to them that is not found in dead, processed foods. You may feel that your connections to the earth, God, and others have deeper meaning, and you may *feel* more. Eating and drinking the rainbow may feel innately right to you. Go with it; explore it more. This is the perfect time to make quiet time for yourself, get centered, and turn off the constant static of life. Meditate, pray, get in the zone, and focus inward to find your inner calm. You need this on a daily basis.

This is the perfect time to make quiet time for yourself, get centered, and turn off the constant static of life.

Supreme Confidence

Look at yourself! You are hot! And many of you are wearing your skinny jeans now! But even if you haven't reached your final weight-loss goal or those skinny jeans don't fit you quite right just yet, keep going. You have made great progress, and you are just bursting with pride! Confidence is the best accessory and a powerful force. They say, "It ain't what they call you; it's what you answer to," and you will be answering to the "OMG, you got hot" comment from someone, for sure. Confidence is beautiful; insecurity is ugly; and when you feel good about yourself, everything changes. This is the foundation of all great success. Don't lose this feeling. Don't go back to your old habits, even if you are having a bad day. You know what to do now. And know you are loved   I love you—and I want you to thrive in your new body and your new natural lifestyle! Hooray for you!

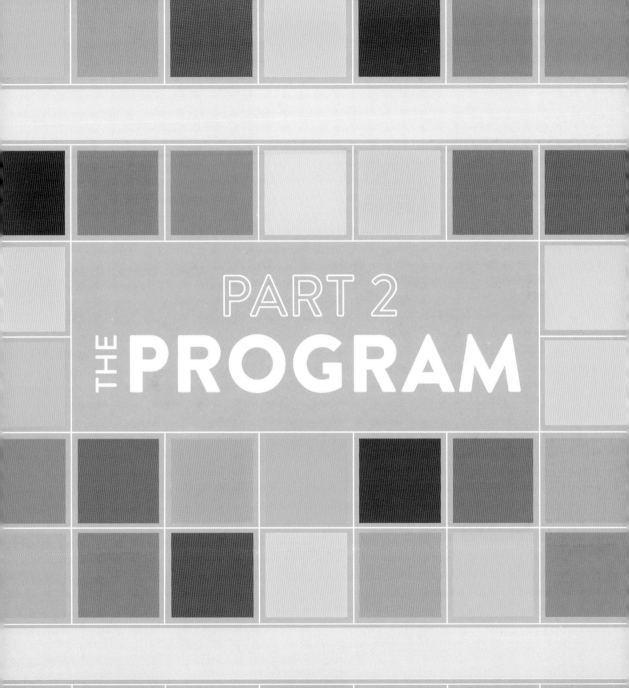

PART 2
THE PROGRAM

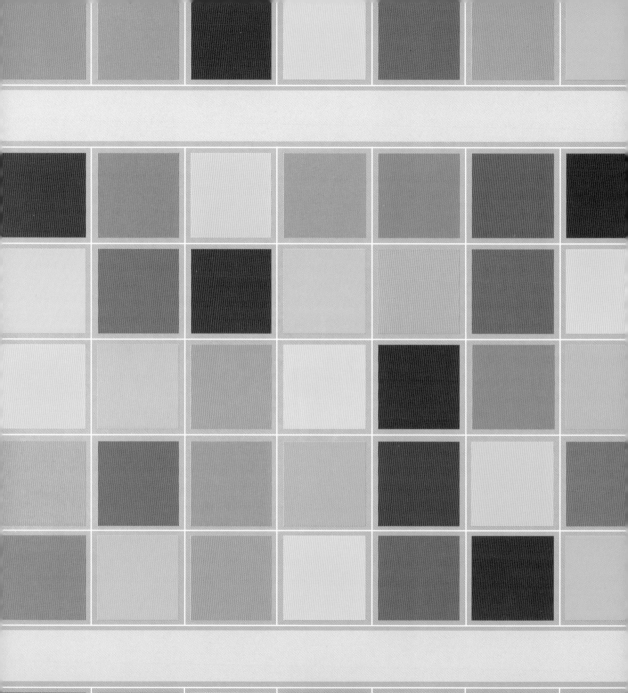

6

THE RAINBOW JUICE CLEANSE PROGRAM

NOW THAT YOU HAVE SOME EDUCATED BACKGROUND information under your belt, it's time to learn the details of the program options and what to do next to get to the end of that rainbow.

● The Weigh-In

Yes, the dreaded weigh-in. You won't, however, dread it in a week. In fact, if you continue to consume the Rainbow Cleanse juices, foods, and recipes, and make them more a part of your lifestyle than the foods you may be currently eating, you will love weigh-in days!

Keep in mind that the scale measures everything—all your muscles, bones, organs, fat, the meal you just ate, the meal you shouldn't have eaten, the meal you are thinking about eating, and even the glass of water you just drank. So each time you weigh yourself, be sure to weigh in at the same time of day, preferably first thing in the morning before you have consumed any food or drink.

Measuring Up with an Unexpected Tool

Your success isn't just about what it says on the scale. Your inches (cm) lost may trump your pounds (kg) lost in measuring your success. Many times, especially if you are exercising, you will see a loss in inches (cm) before you see a loss in pounds (kg). Don't worry: Measuring up doesn't have to require any fancy equipment, not even a tape measure (unless you prefer to take measurements). We are going to perform the "Skinny Jeans Test." Simply pull out those skinny jeans that haven't fit you since your Jane Fonda workout video days and try them on. If that is just too horrifying a thought, pull out that dress you can't seem to squeeze into, even while wearing three sets of Spanx, or try that shirt that splits open and pops off a button every time you button it up and breathe.

Squeeze yourself into that item of clothing, and note how it feels and how it can't button or zip up. Torturous, I know.

> Many times, especially if you are exercising, you will see a loss in inches (cm) before you see a loss in pounds (kg).

Now maybe even take a picture of yourself in that outfit. Oh, come on, it's not that bad! Wait and see what happens in a week and more! This is probably the worst part of the entire program, and now you are done. The next time you put those jeans on, they are going to feel different—and better! I know this step can be incredibly frustrating, but, as alternative-medicine advocate Deepak Chopra, MD, says, "All great changes are preceded by chaos." You will be making some great changes with this program, and clothing can be a very useful and very motivating tool in tracking your weight-loss progress during the cleanse.

Getting with the Program

This is a juice cleanse, a detox, a fast, and for many that may seem a bit daunting. So, for those who have never undertaken a cleanse before or for those who have never gone more than a few hours without satisfying their oral fixation with solid food, I offer two phases to transition yourself into the full-on, seven-day Rainbow Juice Cleanse.

THE TWO-WEEK RAINBOW WARM-UP

If you have a health challenge or are not quite ready to give up your unhealthy food habits all at once, this may be the phase for you. The Rainbow Warm-Up begins the taste-bud transition by introducing the Rainbow Cleanse juices, one each day, but allows you to continue with much of your usual diet. How-ever, it is strongly recommended that you start making posi-tive changes toward a healthier diet during this warm-up period. Here, you are given the option to transi-tion yourself to the cleanse—slowly, over a two-week span—making small or large changes, as you see fit. Now, that doesn't sound so bad, does it?

The idea is for you to make your diges-tive system, your body, your scale, and, most likely, your doctor very happy by starting to eat less from the box and more from the earth. Let's ease into the concept of eating real food, not heavily processed food. Start off simply by incorporating some of the Rainbow foods (page 173) and Rainbow recipes (page 121) in place of

what you are currently eating. But always have one Rainbow Cleanse juice (page 89) each day as a snack, or even—if you dare—a meal replacement. You may or may not lose weight during this learning curve phase (but still do the "Skinny Jeans Test").

Here, we slowly introduce the dietary color concept of the revolutionary Rainbow Cleanse juices, Rainbow Cleanse foods, and Rainbow Cleanse recipes as you start to crave more and more of the rainbow and its magical phytonutri-ents. If you are starting to get hangry, keep in mind that this phase is not necessarily about eating less. When you are hungry, or even hangry, eat. This phase is about eat-ing better, getting away from dead, acidic food, and finally starting to nourish your body at the cellular level.

> Start to eat less from the box and more from the earth.

1 Weigh in and skinny jeans up. Record your findings in a notebook, no matter how shocking or depressing.

2 Give up at least one bad habit each day—soda, coffee, ice cream, fried fish, French fries—whatever vices you are finally ready to abandon. Write down the changes you make over the next two weeks.

3 Start eating more foods from the Rainbow foods list, and preparing them with the least amount of processing possible. Remember, the more processed a food is, the less nutrition it possesses; the more toxins it contains, the more toxic you become; the harder it is to lose weight, the more depressed you become; the more you hit the drive-through, the less likely your fat feet will fit in your Louboutins. Your old ways simply won't open new doors or get you any glamorous new shoes.

4 Incorporate some of the Rainbow food recipes into your daily diet as you taper off the foods that little voice inside your head always tells you you shouldn't be eating. There are delicious recipes for breakfast, lunch, dinner, and snacks to choose from. You can start with dessert, if you must—just start somewhere! You won't feel deprived!

5 Drink one Rainbow Cleanse juice each day. You can choose from the twenty options provided.

6 Stop complaining. If you are reading this book, you know you have to make some changes! Based on twenty years of experience, I know that if you change some of your habits, over time you will end up disliking some of the very food vices you right now consider your favorites. You will develop new favorites. So don't give up: Your stomach shouldn't be a wastebasket. Remember that the difference between try and triumph is a little oomph. So, give yourself a little oomph, and get your booty moving! This is your chance. Go pick out some recipes and eat!

7 If you get hangry, just eat more, but try your best to eat or drink from the Rainbow foods list and the Rainbow recipes.

8 After the two weeks are up, weigh in, skinny jeans up, celebrate, and move on to the Rainbow Rev-Up phase.

Note: Don't go overboard on the fruits, fatty fruits (avocados, olives), nuts, and seeds (and their milks, butters, and cheeses) when transitioning off the Standard American Diet. For many, these are the go-to, healthier, "comfort" foods. Yes, they are healthy and they can certainly be a part of your diet, but you want to try to move more to the greens, sprouts, superfoods, veggies, and veggie juices to achieve optimal health, to curb sugar cravings, to detox, and to promote weight loss.

THE ONE-WEEK RAINBOW REV-UP

If you are starting the Rainbow Rev-Up phase, you have either successfully completed the Rainbow Warm-Up, or you are a daredevil who is ready to cut the cord and ditch your old habits all at once. Either way, I am proud of you!

The Rainbow Rev-Up phase speeds up the transition process quite a bit by utilizing only the Rainbow Cleanse juices for seven days, and also incorporating only the Rainbow Cleanse foods, which are light, phytonutrient-rich, delicious, and full of vibrant color. The Rainbow Cleanse foods allow you to munch on a wide range of scrumptious, colorful, raw, organic, easy-to-digest, health-giving, disease-busting, and weight loss–promoting foods—does it get any better than that? This allows your digestive system to transition off the overly cooked and processed foods you may have been consuming. You can consume breakfast, lunch, dinner, snacks, and desserts from the Rainbow Cleanse foods list and from the scrumptious recipes provided. You can expect to start reaping the weight loss, pH balancing, detoxifying, energy-increasing, and disease-busting benefits in this phase.

On days 1–3, consume only the Rainbow Cleanse foods, recipes, and juices. On day 4, consume only Rainbow Cleanse juice (all day), and then resume the foods and juices on days 5–7. This one-day juice fast in the middle of the week gives the digestive system a rest and helps in transitioning to the Rainbow Juice Cleanse itself. After seven days on the Rainbow Rev-Up, you can completely shift to the full-on, seven-day, all-juice Rainbow Juice Cleanse.

❶ Weigh in and skinny jeans up. Record your findings in a notebook. Be sure to record your weight each day. In addition, keep a daily food and juice journal to track your progress.

❷ Consume at least one Rainbow juice per day. On day 1, start with a red juice; day 2, orange; day 3, yellow; day 4, green; day 5, blue/indigo/violet. You can have more than one juice each day, if you choose, just keep them all the same color during that particular day. On days 6 and 7, you choose what color juice you wish to have that day. You can choose colors you found to be your favorites, but I encourage you to boldly go where no one has gone before and choose a juice you haven't had yet during the week, so as to flood your body with as much varied nutrition as possible. You can drink your juice first thing in the morning to get you going, as a midafternoon pick-me-up, or even as a meal replacement, and you can have more than one a day, if you are feeling adventurous.

❸ The rest of the food you will be consuming throughout the day will come only from the Rainbow foods list or the Rainbow recipes. Pick out foods that appeal to you, but try not to eat the same thing each day. This is not meant to be a restrictive phase, so when you are hungry, eat! Just be sure to stick with a wide variety of unprocessed, nourishing, and very easy-to-digest, blood sugar–stabilizing Rainbow foods and Rainbow recipes. These are designed to detoxify your body and prepare your digestive system for the seven-day Rainbow Juice Cleanse.

❹ If you get hangry, eat! But only from the approved foods, recipes, and juices lists.

❺ Day 4 is your first experiment with an all-day (one-day) juice cleanse. Don't be afraid. You can drink as many juices throughout the day as you desire from the twenty available Rainbow juices, or you can stick with the day 4 green theme. You should not be hungry or hangry. If you are, drink!

❻ To recap, consume Rainbow foods, Rainbow recipes, and Rainbow juices on days 1–3 and days 5–7. Consume only Rainbow juices on day 4.

❼ Weigh in, skinny jeans up, and celebrate!

❽ Once you've completed the seven-day Rainbow Rev-Up, it's off to the seven-day Rainbow Juice Cleanse!

● The Seven-Day Rainbow Juice Cleanse

Congratulations! You have either worked your way up to this final phase, or you are just ready to jump in feet first. Regardless, you are about to embark on an exciting seven-day cleansing journey. I love your spirited nature! You are all-in!

During the Rainbow Juice Cleanse, you will be consuming only phytonutrient-loaded, low-glycemic Rainbow Cleanse juices for seven days, and you will reap the rainbow of benefits. Drink one color of the rainbow each day to supercharge your body with the predominant phytonutrient family of that day's juice color. Consume only Rainbow Cleanse foods and recipes four days before beginning this phase to allow the digestive

> The Rainbow Cleanse helps to detoxify your body, combat disease, banish the signs of aging, gain energy, and achieve the ultimate in weight loss.

system to transition away from cooked and/or processed foods. Your body needs light and easily digestible foods to ease into and out of the full-on juice cleanse.

You will consume the Rainbow foods and recipes for four days after the cleanse, as well, to ease back onto solid foods. The Rainbow rewards kick in full force during this cleanse, unveiling the pot of gold: detoxifying your body, combating disease, banishing the signs of aging, gaining a surfeit of energy, and achieving the ultimate in weight loss—reaching your seven-pound goal in seven days. If you follow a healthy diet and/or have performed cleanses in the past, I encourage you to jump right in to the seven-day Rainbow Juice Cleanse phase.

THE RAINBOW JUICE CLEANSE

1 Weigh in and skinny jeans up. Record your findings in a notebook.

2 For four days, consume only Rainbow foods and Rainbow recipes to ease your digestive system into the program. These four days are not considered part of the seven-day Rainbow Cleanse.

3 Weigh in on day 1. Record your findings.

4 **DAYS 1–5:** Consume the following color juices all day:

DAY 1: RED
DAY 2: ORANGE
DAY 3: YELLOW
DAY 4: GREEN
DAY 5: BLUE/INDIGO/VIOLET

Each day, all day, drink the same color juice; choose from any or all of the four juice recipes provided for each color, and drink as much as you want throughout the day. (Note: Most people drink four to seven servings of juice per day, but it may vary for you. If you get hungry, drink a juice.)

5 **DAYS 6 AND 7:** You choose the juices you would like to drink. You can drink an entire day of all one color or drink a variety of colors throughout the two days.

6 Congratulations! The juice cleanse is complete! Feel free to weigh in and skinny jeans up, but be sure to consume only Rainbow foods and Rainbow recipes for the next four days to ease your digestive system back into digesting solid, easy-to-digest foods.

7 Weigh in, skinny jeans up, and celebrate again!

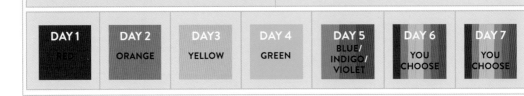

DAY 1	DAY 2	DAY 3	DAY 4	DAY 5	DAY 6	DAY 7
RED	ORANGE	YELLOW	GREEN	BLUE/INDIGO/VIOLET	YOU CHOOSE	YOU CHOOSE

After the Cleanse and Over the Rainbow

If you love your new transformation—don't stop! You have invested in your hot little self this far, and you are on the right track! The Rainbow Juice Cleanse foods, recipes, and juices are a very healthy way of living. In fact, you can do this cleanse again in another six months. In the meantime, you can even do what many healing centers advise: Cleanse one day a week with nothing but fresh, organic juices. You can also incorporate juices each day along with all the healthy foods and recipes. Don't lose the progress you just gained!

Now that you have lost weight, booted the sugar cravings, and feel totally in control, focus on losing the mind-set and the unhealthy lifestyle that got you there in the first place. Your new healthy habits can be just as addicting as your old ones, but with much better side effects: more energy, great health, glowing skin, and don't forget that feeling when you were able to slide into those skinny jeans. Not much feels better than that. This is what it feels like to be over the rainbow! Being truly healthy is not about constantly counting calories and feeling hangry and deprived; it's about cleansing and then nourishing your body with real food, as untainted by food manufacturers as possible, so you are energized, satiated, feeling confident, and ready to take life's bull by the horns! Isn't that what life is all about, anyway?

Here are some additional tips to help you on your Rainbow journey:

Juice those leafy greens. When juicing leafy greens, you quickly discover that they spin through your juicer (particularly in a centrifugal juicer), oftentimes without even juicing. The trick is to roll a handful of the leaves (spinach, romaine, etc.) into a tight ball and then push it through, so the juicer has something to "catch" as it juices.

Note: Leafy greens work very well in a blender when making the smoothies in this book.

> Your new healthy habits can be just as addicting as your old ones, but with much better side effects.

Consume at least thirty-two ounces each day for optimal health. In order to get the most from your juicing, you need to infuse your body with enough juice, especially during the cleanse. Don't just make six or eight ounces (177–236 ml) and call it a day. Instead, work up to consuming a minimum of thirty-two ounces (946 ml) of juice throughout the day.

Understand your tainted taste buds. If you've been eating the Standard American Diet for a while, your taste buds have become accustomed to sugary, salty, and chemically enhanced foods. So your initial sip of a veggie juice may taste a bit odd. Stick with it. Once you cleanse your body and detoxify it of all chemical and synthetic additives, your taste buds will bounce back to life, and you will once again appreciate all of nature's foods as you were meant to!

Use a straw. In the beginning, you may find it best to use a straw to drink your juice. Again, those tainted taste buds play tricks on your innate tendencies to crave nature's foods, but this will subside and before long you will be chewing your juice.

Chew your juice. Once your taste buds have reset and you don't feel you need a straw to drink your juice, swish it around in your mouth and chew your juice—yes, chew—to stimulate the enzyme salivary amylase to begin the digestive process. Carbohydrate digestion begins in the mouth, and this will aid in adequate digestion.

Drink your juice soon after it's made. Due to the oxidation process, which causes a loss of nutrients, it is best to consume your juice fresh and not long after you make it. We all know that when we slice open an apple and don't eat it immediately, it turns brown. This is the oxidation process in action. This also happens to your fresh-made Rainbow juice, although it's harder to tell because the juice is a vibrant color. My good friend Lenore Vassil likes to tell her disciples to "drink your green juice within fifteen minutes, or it loses its magic."

> The oxidation process causes a loss of nutrients, so it is best to consume your juice fresh.

Store your juice properly. If you cannot drink all your juice right after making it or if you are making a big batch to use throughout the day, be sure to store the juice in an airtight container, filling it all the way to the top. That way, no oxygen can get in. This will help to minimize oxidation. Then store it in the refrigerator.

Try some juice-boosting extras. Increase the nutrition of your juices even more by adding a juice-boosting extra (see pages 62-65).

Reuse the fiber. The fiber that comes out of the end of your juicer can be reused in various ways and does not need to be thrown out. You can compost it, mix it into your dog's food (dogs need fiber, too), or do what my friend Chef Terry Botel (author of *Vegan Up*) from Switzerland does, and add it to soups, salads, or other recipes (for example, use carrot pulp in raw carrot cake). Keep in mind that if you are using a low-end juicer, these often do not have the power to "pull" as much juice from the produce as the higher-end models. So you may want to rejuice the pulp several times if it feels wet to extract as much juice from it as possible.

Juice in your workplace. I have worked with countless clients who juice at the workplace. Many companies have a breakroom and will purchase a juicer for their employees to use while at work. Just bring your own organic veggies with you, and your new daily juicing routine won't be interrupted. You may even inspire your coworkers to forgo the coffee and juice with you.

Juice when traveling. With a little preplanning, it is still possible to keep up with your juicing routine while you're traveling so you don't feel tempted to buy pasteurized juice. Go online and scope out the local health food stores in the area you will be visiting, as well as healthy restaurants. In some cities, you will see "raw food" restaurants that will know exactly what a raw veggie juice is and will be happy to serve you theirs.

Another great way to keep up your juicing regimen while traveling is with organic green powders. These are organic greens that have been dehydrated and blended into a fine powder. You can purchase these at your local health food store. Simply mix a spoonful of green powder in a glass of filtered water, stir, and drink. Many of my clients keep a container of green powder in their desk drawer at work for a quick pick-me-up snack when there is no time for lunch or real juicing.

Juice when dining out. Dining out during any of the phases of the Rainbow Juice Cleanse is not difficult; it just requires a little extra thought—and your health is worth it! Here are some tips to help you keep up with the program while dining out:

1 Try to choose a restaurant with a varied menu and one you know will have the right options for you. Regardless of where you go, stick to the approved foods list (pages 174–80). You know what you should be eating. Just do it!

2 Plan ahead. Check out the restaurant's menu online, so you know ahead of time what you will order.

3 Make a special request. I do this often. You are always safe with a large veggie salad. Ask the waiter to make a big bowl of greens with all the veggies they have in the kitchen—I call it the "Kitchen Sink Salad." They are usually happy to accommodate.

4 Watch out for dressings and sauces. This is where dining out can rain on your rainbow. Avoid creamy dressings and sauces, as well as toppings like bacon bits and (fried) croutons. You can ask for an orange or a lime and squeeze the juices over your salad or even bring your own dressing or sea veggies to add to the salad.

5 Order several veggie side dishes or a veggie-based soup, but ask the chef not to add salt.

6 Wear your skinny jeans or an item of clothing that either fits you just right or may be a little snug or form-fitting. This may prevent you from overeating, especially if you go to an all-you-can-eat restaurant.

PART 3
THE RAINBOW
RECIPES AND APPROVED FOODS

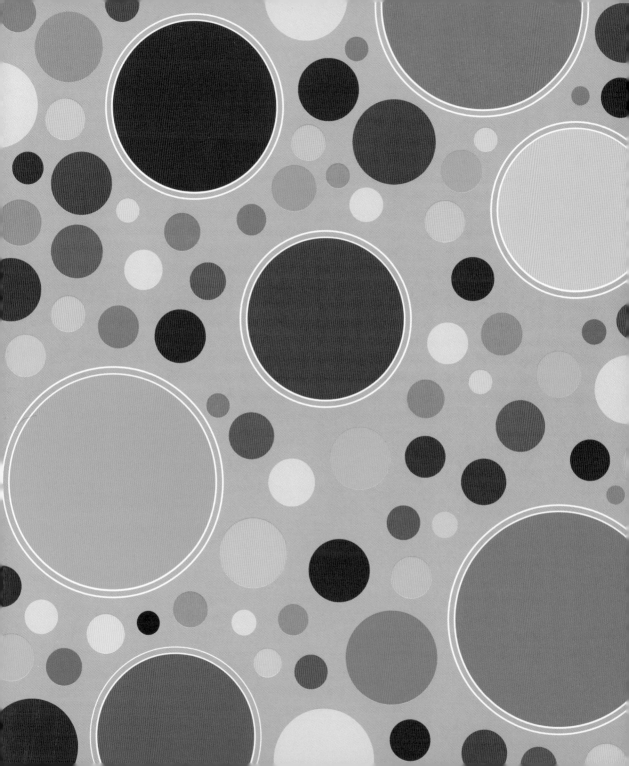

7

JUICES

ALL THE RAINBOW CLEANSE JUICES in this chapter require a juicer, unless otherwise indicated. If this is your first time making veggie juices, and you feel they are too strong for your Standard American Diet–programmed taste buds, you can dilute them by adding a milder-tasting cucumber to the mix or even filtered water. You can also add some lemon, lime, or stevia to sweeten them. Or just stick a straw in it and suck it down within twenty minutes of making it, and let it do its magic!

Note: Juicing the rind of citrus fruits is totally acceptable; in fact, some studies have shown that antioxidants in citrus peels are twenty times more powerful than the juice. But, for some, the oils can be tough on the stomach. So perhaps try half the peel and see how you respond, and only juice the rind if you are using an organic lemon or lime (which you should be). Here we go!

A Taste of Italy

Flush your body with a taste of Italy, and bathe your cells in heart-protective phytonutrients and loads of vitamins A and C, as you savor the flavors and aromas of the Old Country. Load up on more cilantro if you like the taste; it's a whole-body detoxifier.

SERVES 1

4 large tomatoes, sliced in half

2 red bell peppers, cored and seeded

½ handful parsley

½ handful cilantro

½ handful oregano

¼ small onion, peeled

2 garlic cloves (or to taste), peeled

After juicing:

Dulse and kelp flakes, to taste

Stevia, to taste (optional)

Juice all the ingredients. Pour into a glass, add the dulse and kelp flakes and stevia (if desired), and "*cin cin*"!

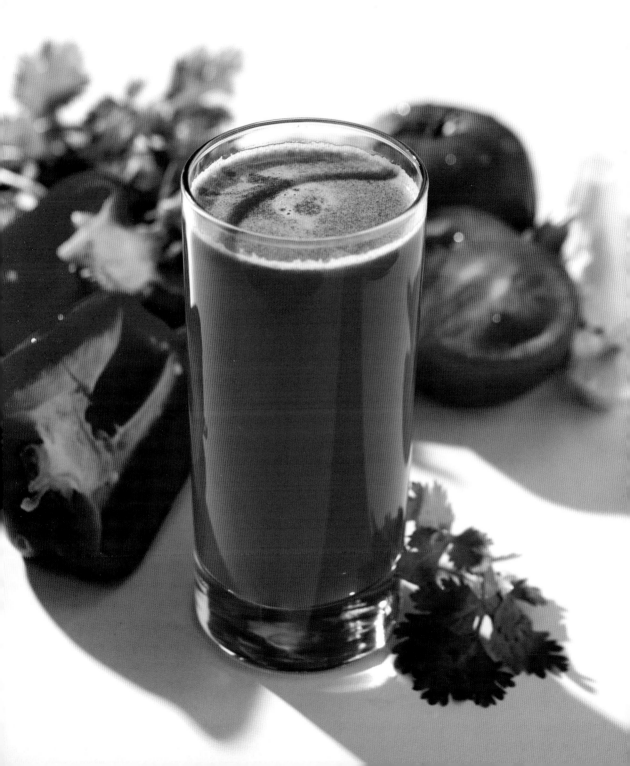

Apple Cider Lime Tonic

No juicer needed with this healing tonic made from raw, unpasteurized, fermented apples, proven to lower blood glucose levels. This tonic also includes lime juice for a big shot of easily absorbable vitamin C and flavonol glycosides, shown to stop cell division in various cancers. You will definitely feel its energizing effects!

SERVES 1

- 1 cup (200 ml) filtered water, very cold, or 1 cup (200 ml) coconut water
- 2 teaspoons (10 ml) apple cider vinegar, raw, organic, and unpasteurized (I like Bragg's)
- Juice from two limes (squeezed by hand)

Pour cold, filtered water into a large glass, add the apple cider vinegar, and add about half the lime juice. Give it a taste test. If you are satisfied, drink up; otherwise, add the rest of the lime juice and enjoy!

Rhubarb Gingerade

Tart rhubarb is packed with vitamin K and bioavailable calcium, necessary for healthy bone growth, along with vitamin C and vitamin A. It's known to help lower the bad cholesterol. The potent compounds called gingerols, found in the gingerroot, are known for relieving arthritis pain and overall inflammation.

SERVES 1

1 stalk red rhubarb, roughly chopped (Note: Do *not* juice the leaves. Choose ripe, deeply colored stalks.)

½ head red cabbage, roughly chopped

1½ inch (4 cm) fresh gingerroot, unpeeled

After juicing:

Fresh mint leaves, crushed

Stevia, to taste (optional)

Juice the rhubarb, red cabbage, and gingerroot. Then add the mint. Add stevia, if desired, and enjoy the pleasant pucker!

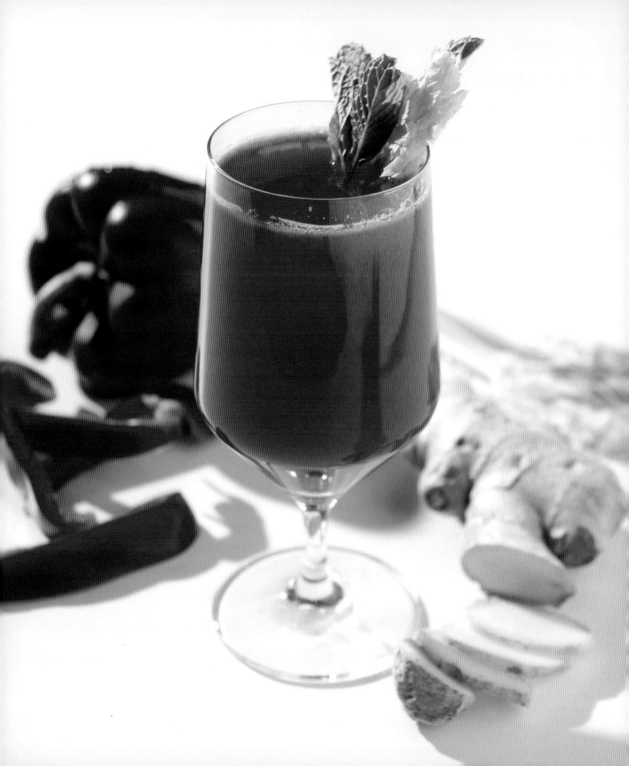

Red Pepper-Mint Juice

Restore and rejuvenate yourself with this soothing, minty juice, containing vitamin E, manganese, and over thirty known members of the carotenoid phytonutrient family! Impressive!

SERVES 1

- 2 red bell peppers, cored and seeded
- 2 stalks celery, roughly chopped
- 1 inch (2.5 cm) fresh gingerroot, unpeeled

After juicing:

Fresh mint leaves, crushed

Stevia, to taste (optional)

Run the red peppers, celery, and gingerroot through the juicer. Pour the juice in a glass along with a crunched up handful of mint and add stevia, if desired.

Autumn Sunrise

Awaken your groggy eyes in the morning with this mild but sweet and vibrant juice. It harnesses anti-inflammatory carotenoids and immune-boosting vitamins C, A, and B$_6$.

SERVES 1

2 orange bell peppers, cored and seeded

1 large cucumber, cut into chunks

After juicing:

Dried cilantro

Stevia, to taste (optional)

Juice the peppers and cucumber. Pour into a glass and then add cilantro and stevia, if desired.

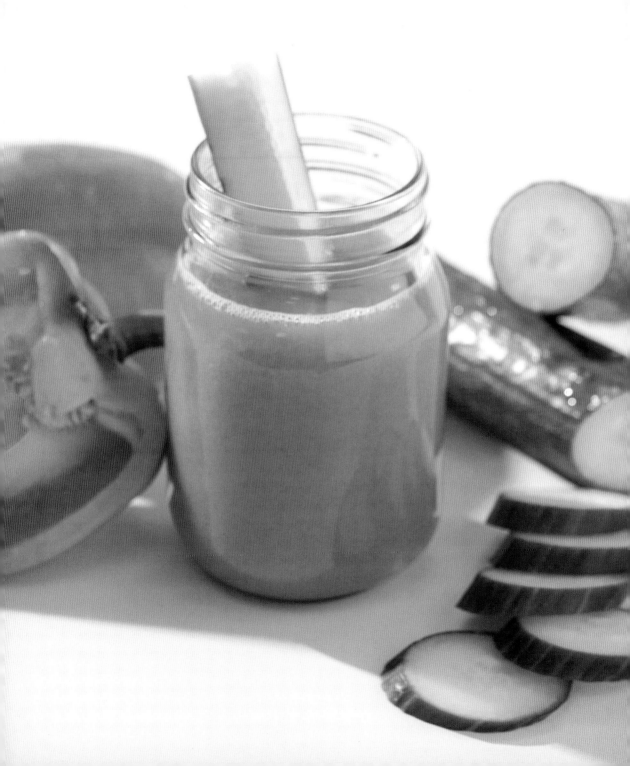

Cinnamon Pumpkin Pie

Fragrant and sweet, this juice is loaded with potassium, pantothenic acid, magnesium, vitamin C, and alpha- and beta-carotene from the pumpkin. Cinnamon contributes high manganese, plus anticlotting, anti-inflammatory, blood sugar–stabilizing, and triglyceride-lowering effects.

SERVES 1

2 cups (400 ml) chopped
   pumpkin pulp

¼ teaspoon (1.3 ml)
   ground ginger or
   2 inches (5 cm) fresh
   gingerroot, unpeeled

After juicing:

¼ teaspoon (1.3 ml)
   ground cinnamon

Stevia, to taste

Juice the pumpkin pulp and gingerroot, and pour into a glass. Add cinnamon and stevia.

Minty Pepper Orange Juice

This simple yet refreshing drink is loaded with over thirty different members of the phytonutrient carotenoid family, as well as vitamins A and C.

SERVES 1

3 orange bell peppers, cored and seeded

1 head white endive, cut into chunks

After juicing:

Fresh mint leaves, crushed

Juice the peppers and endive, and pour into a glass. Add the mint leaves, and enjoy!

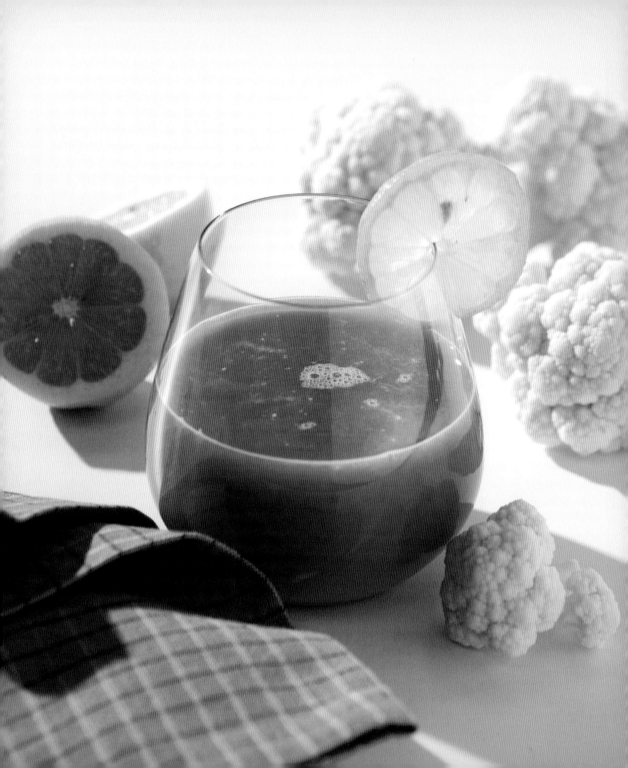

Indian Spiced Cauliflower

Loaded with the phytonutrient glucosinolate from the cruciferous cauliflower and potent anti-inflammatory, anticancer properties of the turmeric, this natural liver and kidney cleanser is also packed with debris-digesting enzymes for excellent cleansing support. Don't forget the pepper; the piperine in it is needed to help increase the absorption of the turmeric.

SERVES 1

1 head cauliflower, cut into chunks

¼ lemon

1 inch (2.5 cm) fresh gingerroot, unpeeled

2 inches (5 cm) turmeric root, unpeeled, or 1 teaspoon (5 ml) turmeric powder

After juicing:

Black pepper, to taste

Coriander, to taste

Cumin, to taste

Juice the cauliflower, lemon, and gingerroot. Add the turmeric root as well, or if using turmeric powder, add it to the finished juice. Pour the juice into a glass, and sprinkle in desired amounts of the black pepper, coriander, and cumin.

Thai One on Tonic

Topped off with the delicate and refreshing flavor of lemongrass, this zucchini-based juice is packed with lutein and zeaxanthin, which support the eyes against age-related macular degeneration and cataracts. It's also packed with many of the B vitamins, zinc, magnesium, and omega-3s, which promote healthy sugar metabolism, helping with blood sugar stabilization.

SERVES 1

½ head cauliflower, cut into chunks

2 zucchini or yellow summer squash, cut into chunks

1 inch (2.5 cm) fresh gingerroot, unpeeled

After Juicing:

1½ teaspoons (7.5 ml) very finely grated lemongrass

Fresh basil leaf

Juice the cauliflower, zucchini, and gingerroot, and pour into a glass. Garnish with lemongrass and basil.

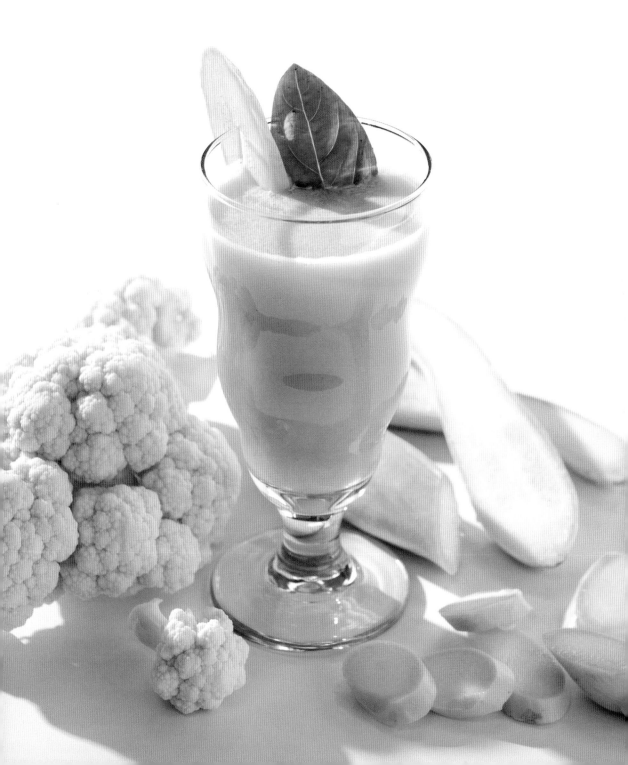

Cha Cha Cha Chia Summer Delight

Chia seeds are prized for their energy-sustaining, anti-inflammatory, detoxi-fying and high-protein properties, as well as for being high in omega-3s. This juice is also bursting with the antioxidants vitamin C and manganese, known for helping the body produce healthy collagen and essential for wound healing.

SERVES 1

2 zucchini or yellow
summer squash, cut
into chunks

½ lemon

After juicing:

2 teaspoons (10 ml)
chia seeds

Stevia, to taste

Juice the zucchini and lemon. Pour the juice into a glass, and add the chia seeds and stevia. Stir and enjoy.

Pot of Yellow Pepper Gold

You've reached the pot of gold with this juice. Loaded with vitamins A, B, and C; magnesium, copper, potassium, and manganese; and phytonutrients like zea-xanthin, beta-cryptoxanthin, and lutein, it's satisfying to both your taste buds and your blood sugar, as well as beneficial to your eye and retinal health.

SERVES 1

1 yellow winter squash, cut into chunks

3 yellow bell peppers, cored and seeded

1 inch (2.5 cm) fresh gingerroot, unpeeled

After juicing:

Juice from two limes (squeezed by hand)

Juice the squash, peppers, and gingerroot. Pour into a glass, and add the lime juice.

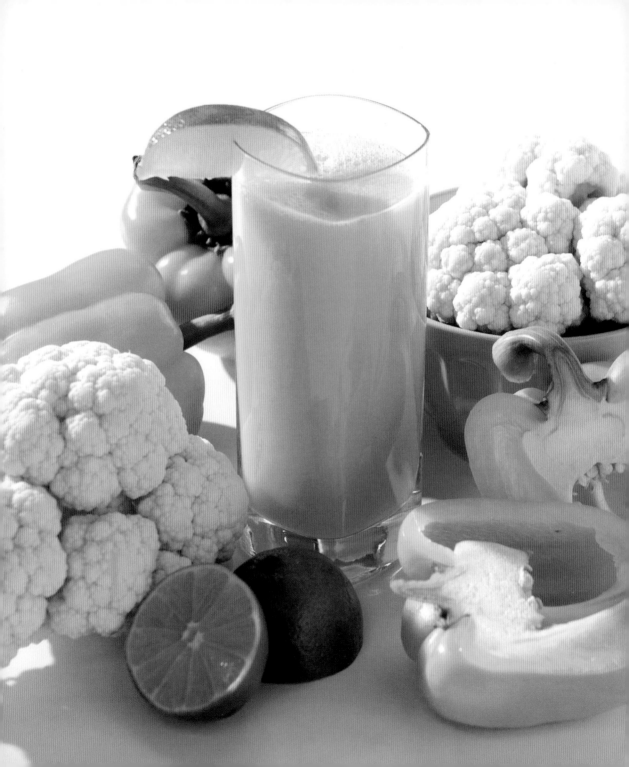

Creamed Yellow Pepper

Loaded with vitamin K, one of the hallmark anti-inflammatory nutrients, as well as omega-3s, vitamins C and E, and heart-healthy phytonutrients, this juice offers great cardiovascular support, keeping the arteries clean and the blood flowing!

SERVES 1

1 head cauliflower, chopped into chunks

2 yellow bell peppers, cored and seeded

1 lime

Juice the cauliflower, peppers, and lime (rind on lime is optional). Pour into a glass, and enjoy.

Cabbage Patch Greens

Made with spinach, one of the top nutrient-rich greens, and cucumber, whose alkalizing and detoxifying properties are well known, this juice is also filled with some of the most powerful antioxidants found in cruciferous veggies, thanks to its ulcer-relieving, bad cholesterol–lowering green cabbage and broccoli.

SERVES 1

¼ wedge green cabbage, cut into chunks

2 stalks broccoli, cut into chunks

1 cucumber, cut into chunks

Large handful spinach leaves

Small handful parsley

Small handful basil leaves

Juice the cabbage, broccoli, and cucumber. Roll the spinach, parsley, and basil into a ball and run them through the juicer. Pour into a glass, and drink up.

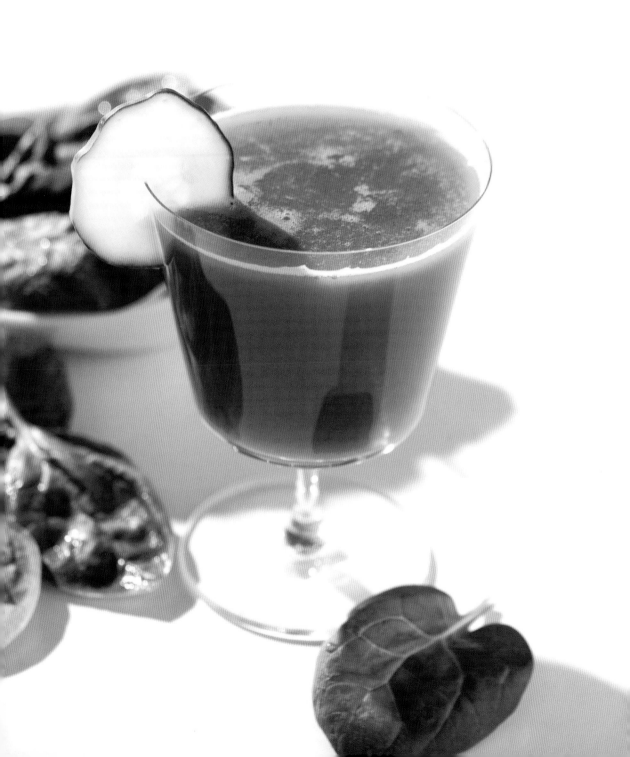

Kale Lemon Aid

Light and refreshing, this lemonade features kale, the queen of greens, and is jam-packed with highly absorbable anticancer phytonutrients; vitamins A, C, and K; the minerals copper, potassium, iron, and manganese; and sun-kissed chlorophyll.

SERVES 1

1 head green endive, cut into chunks

1 cucumber, cut into chunks

5 green kale leaves

¼ lemon with the peel

2 inches (5 cm) fresh gingerroot, unpeeled

After Juicing:

Lemon slice

Juice the endive and cucumber. Roll the kale leaves into a ball so the juicer has something to catch, and run them through the juicer. Juice the lemon and gingerroot. Garnish the finished juice with a lemon slice, and knock it back!

Green Fennel Cooler

This juice contains very light and cleansing ingredients that are full of vitamin C, beta-carotene, and folate, as well as electrolytes like potassium and phosphorus. The fennel greens, known to reduce water retention and ease stomach cramps, contain the oil anethole, which gives this juice a really refreshing aftertaste.

SERVES 1

1 cucumber, cut into chunks

½ green zucchini, cut into chunks

½ yellow summer squash, cut into chunks

Large bunch fennel greens

Juice all the ingredients, pour into a glass, and lap it up.

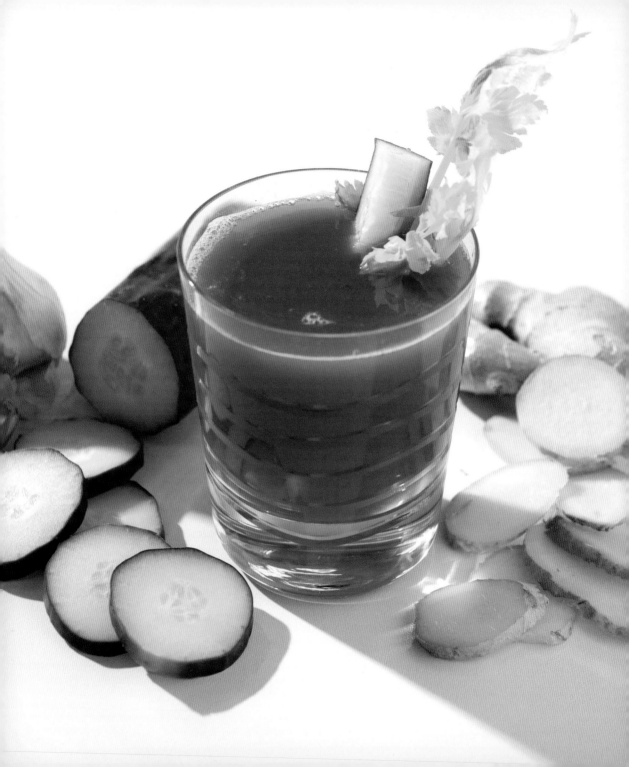

Hippocrates Health Institute's Famous Green Juice

My favorite juice of all time—and an alkaline nutritional powerhouse at that!—this juice delivers the right hook to a toxic body. The high-protein sprouts are more nutritious than your most nourishing veggies, so enjoy them in this juice and add them to others for extra nutrients. Add the garlic and/or ginger for added nutritional properties.

SERVES 1 (BIG GULP SIZE)

3 stalks celery, roughly chopped

1½ cucumbers, cut into chunks

2 cups (400 ml) sunflower sprouts

2 cups (400 ml) pea green sprouts

Juice from 1 garlic clove, peeled, or 1 inch (2.5 cm) fresh gingerroot, unpeeled (optional)

Juice all the ingredients and sip it down!

Minty Mauve Cabbage Magic

Packed with aromatic, stomach-soothing mint and blood pressure–regulating celery, this juice gets its oomph from the gentle, cleansing, and intestinal-healing properties of the purple cabbage. The vibrantly colored cabbage is loaded with anticancer phytonutrients and vitamins A, B_1, B_2, B_6, C, E, and K, plus folate.

SERVES 1

4 purple cabbage leaves

2 stalks celery, roughly chopped

1 bunch fresh mint leaves

½ small lime (or more, to taste)

Chop the cabbage leaves into smaller pieces and juice them along with the celery, mint leaves, and lime. Pour into a glass, and enjoy.

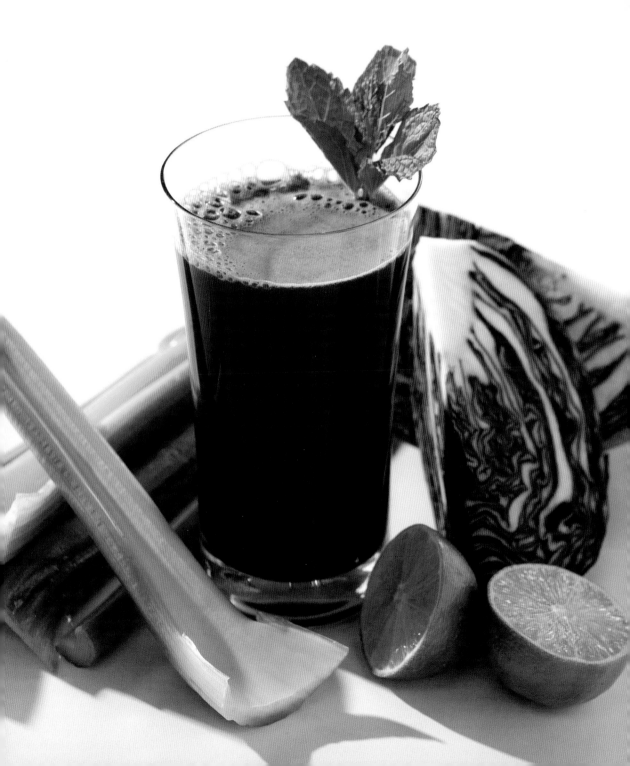

Purple Sea Asparagus

Slightly sweeter than green asparagus, purple asparagus brings on the super-nutrition in this juice, along with the mineral-loaded sea veggies dulse and kelp, known for their high mineral content and bone-building properties.

SERVES 1

1 bunch purple asparagus

1 lemon

After juicing:

Dulse and kelp flakes, to taste

Stevia, to taste

Juice the asparagus and lemon, and pour into a glass. Add dulse and kelp flakes and stevia, as desired.

Purple Punch

Light, refreshing, and polyphenol-rich, this juice gives a big antioxidant knock-out punch to cancer, heart disease, premature aging, and toxic heavy metals.

SERVES 1

1 head purple Belgian
  endive, cut into chunks

1 cucumber, cut into
  chunks

After juicing:

Dulse and kelp flakes,
  to taste

Juice the endive and cucumber. Add dulse and kelp flakes, stir it up, and imbibe.

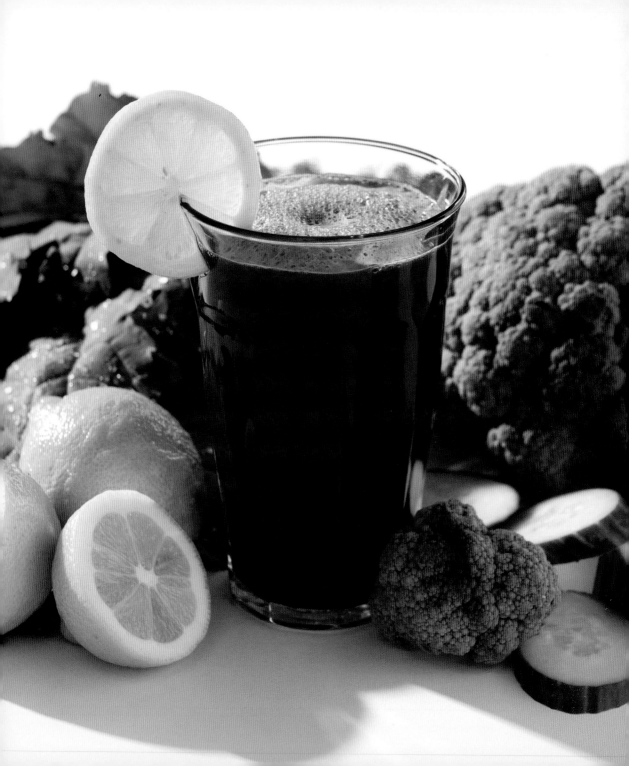

Purple Lemonade

A big star in the kale family, the purple kale in this juice has beneficial antho-cyanin phytonutrient properties, which protect against the oxidative stress of various toxins. A great addition to your cleanse!

SERVES 1

1 head purple cauliflower, cut into chunks

4 purple kale leaves

1 cucumber, cut into chunks

½ lemon

After juicing:

Stevia, to taste

Juice the cauliflower. Roll the kale leaves into a ball, and juice them along with the cucumber and lemon. Pour into a glass, and add stevia.

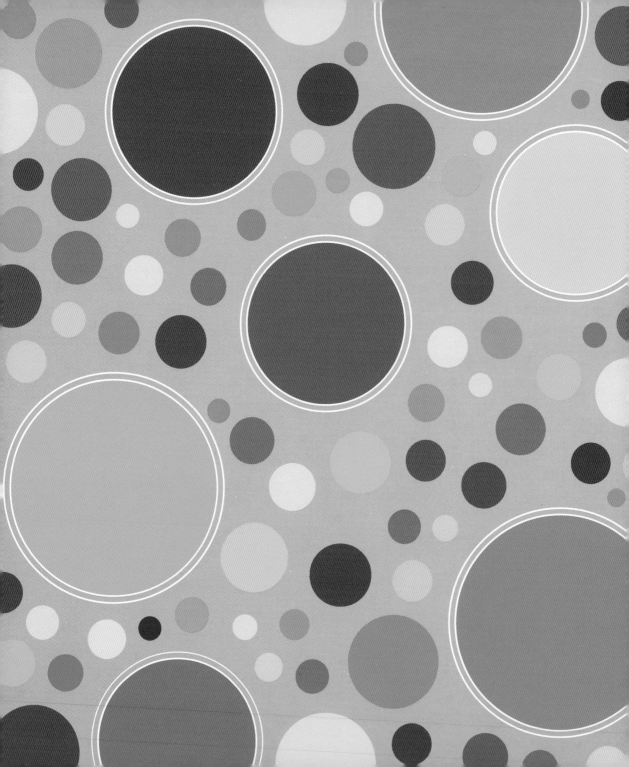

8

SMOOTHIES

PULL OUT YOUR BLENDER and get ready to whip up some nutritious and delicious health-giving smoothies!

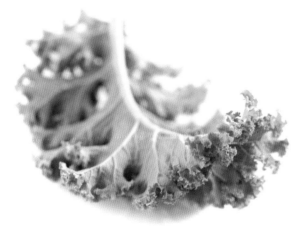

Cinnamon Zucchini Smoothie

Creamy and filling, this low-GI zucchini (fruit) smoothie with a zing of cinnamon is delicious! You can even add a little unsweetened carob powder for a little chocolaty taste.

SERVES 1

½ cup (100 ml) filtered water

2 cups (400 ml) chopped zucchini

1 tablespoon (15 ml) alcohol-free vanilla extract or ground vanilla bean

1 tablespoon (15 ml) ground cinnamon, plus more for dusting

Stevia, to taste

Place all ingredients in a blender, and pulse until silky-smooth. Pour mixture into a glass, sprinkle a dusting of cinnamon on top, and enjoy!

Green Cilantro Smoothie

The ultimate low-calorie, high-nutrient green detox smoothie.

Juice from one lime, (squeezed by hand)

2 cups (400 ml) filtered water

1 cup (200 ml) kale or spinach leaves

1 cup (200 ml) chopped fresh pineapple

½ cup (100 ml) fresh cilantro

½ inch (1.3 cm) fresh gingerroot, unpeeled

1 cup (200 ml) ice

Place all ingredients in the blender, pulse, and enjoy!

Minty Spirulina Kiwi Smoothie

Mean, green, and refreshing, this high-protein spirulina smoothie is sure to get your cells primed and ready for cleansing. The kiwi skin contains vitamin C and fiber, so I never peel them before using.

SERVES 1

1 cup (200 ml) filtered water

3 kiwis, halved, unpeeled

1 cucumber

5 fresh mint leaves

1 tablespoon (15 ml) chia seeds

1 tablespoon (15 ml) spirulina

Place the filtered water, kiwis, cucumber, and mint in the blender, and pulse. Pour in a glass. Add the chia seeds and spirulina. Stir, and imbibe.

9

SHAKES

IF YOU LIKE NUT BUTTERS, YOU WILL LOVE these filling, high-plant-protein, dairy-free, hormone-free, and cholesterol-free shakes. Soak the nuts (and all seeds) in water overnight or for a few hours before using them to soak off the enzyme inhibitors and make them more easily digestible. Pull out your blender, and get shakin'!

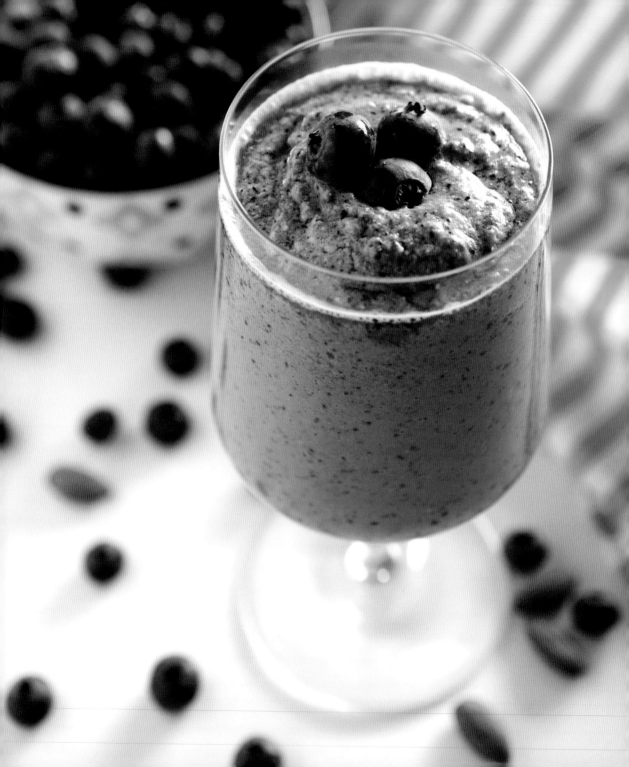

Blueberry Almond Shake

Cool, creamy, and filling, this shake uses phytonutrient-rich blueberries and heart-protecting, high-protein, vitamin E–loaded almonds.

SERVES 1

¾ cup (150 ml) almonds

2 cups (400 ml) filtered water

1 cup (200 ml) fresh blueberries, plus more for garnish

Soak the almonds in water for a few hours or overnight. Drain the liquid and discard. Place the almonds, filtered water, and blueberries in a blender. Pulse and drink.

Cinnamon Walnut Shake

High in omega-3 fatty acids and the highest antioxidant profile of all nuts, the buttery-tasting walnuts in this recipe won't disappoint. Add to that the blood sugar–stabilizing and metabolism-boosting cinnamon, and you've got yourself a shake!

SERVES 1

1 cup (200 ml) walnuts

2 cups (400 ml) filtered
water

1 tablespoon (15 ml)
ground cinnamon

Soak the walnuts in water for a few hours or overnight. Drain the liquid and discard. Place the walnuts and filtered water in a blender and pulse until smooth. Add cinnamon and pulse again.

Pumpkin Pie Shake

Bright orange and festive-tasting, this fiber-filled pumpkin, cinnamon, and nutmeg shake will bring on that holiday feeling, in a healthy way, any time of year.

SERVES 1

¼ cup (50 ml) pumpkin seeds

2 cups (400 ml) filtered water

1 cup (200 ml) pumpkin pulp, skinned and seeded

1 teaspoon (5 ml) alcohol-free vanilla extract or ground vanilla bean

¼ teaspoon (1.3 ml) ground cinnamon

¼ teaspoon (1.3 ml) ground nutmeg

1 teaspoon (5 ml) chia seeds

Soak the pumpkin seeds in water for a few hours or overnight. Discard the liquid, and pour the seeds into a blender with the filtered water. Slice up the pumpkin and add the pulp to the blender. Add vanilla, cinnamon, and nutmeg and pulse. Add chia seeds to the mixture and give one or two pulses to the blender, then pour in a glass, and lap it up.

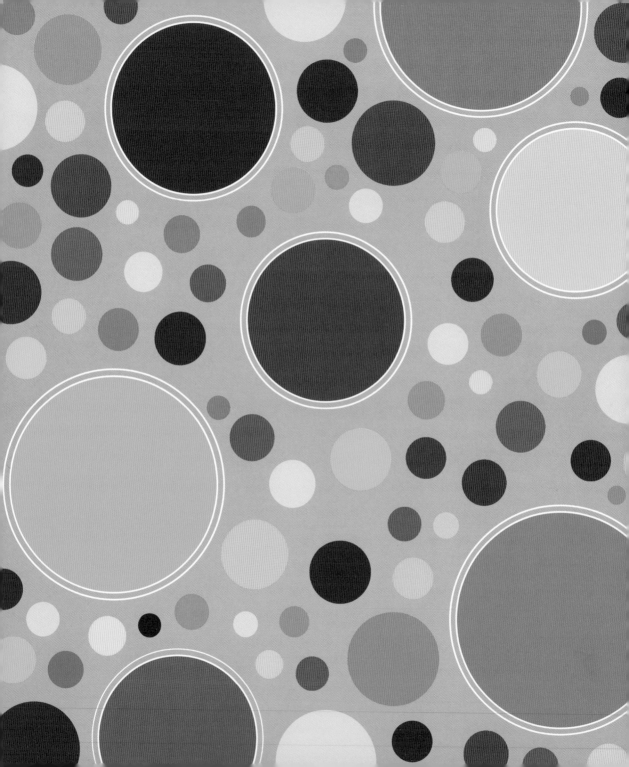

CHAPTER
10
SOUPS

NO SOUP FOR YOU! WELL, NOT IN THIS CASE. For you, delish, cleansing, alkaline, nourishing soups inspired by nature's gardens. These are a great first food after the seven-day Rainbow Juice Cleanse to break the fast. Keep in mind, these are no-cook soups, intended to harness and not destroy the full bounty of enzymes, vitamins, minerals, and phytonutrients found in the ingredients. If you decide to heat them, use a very low setting. Some blenders will even slightly warm as you purée if you leave them running for a few minutes. Even better, just warm up the water used in your soup in a tea kettle (not the microwave), or put your soup bowl in the warming drawer or oven for a few minutes, then pour in your raw soup.

Creamy Basil Asparagus Soup

The creaminess of pine nuts, the pepperiness of basil, and the earthy tones of the fresh asparagus will make you go back for seconds.

SERVES 1

2 cups (400 ml) filtered water

2 bunches asparagus

Handful fresh basil leaves

¼ cup (50 ml) pine nuts (do not need soaking)

1 garlic clove, peeled

1 tablespoon (15 ml) Namo Shoyu or Tamari

For garnish:

Basil sprig

Lemon zest

Turmeric powder

Place all the ingredients in a blender and pulse until creamy. Pour into a bowl. Garnish with a sprig of basil, some lemon zest, and a sprinkle of turmeric powder.

Cream of Curry Cauliflower Soup

Begin your love affair with curry in this smooth, nutrition-packed soup. With up to twenty spices, herbs, and seeds that are pulverized to make curry, you can imagine the goodness you are getting with each sprinkle!

SERVES 1

½ cup (100 ml) almonds

2 cups (400 ml) small cauliflower chunks

2 cups (400 ml) filtered water

½ cup (100 ml) peeled and chopped sweet onion

1 tablespoon (15 ml) chickpea miso

1 garlic clove, peeled

1 tablespoon (15 ml) curry powder, plus more for garnish

Soak the almonds in water for a few hours or overnight. Discard the liquid, and place the almonds in a blender. Add the cauliflower, filtered water, onion, miso, garlic, and curry powder. Pulse until creamy, and pour into a bowl. Garnish with a sprinkle of curry powder.

Minty Cucumber Soup

Mint, cucumber, and scallions conspire with the nut or seed milk of your choice to produce a delicious, cleansing soup.

SERVES 1

1 cucumber, cut into chunks, unpeeled

1 cup (200 ml) nut or seed milk of your choice

½ cup (100 ml) fresh mint leaves

2 tablespoons (30 ml) finely sliced scallions

For garnish:

4 cucumber slices

3 fresh mint leaves

Place all the ingredients in a blender and blend until smooth. Pour into a bowl. Garnish with the cucumber slices and mint leaves.

Spinach and the Sea Soup

This almost instant energy–giving, phytonutrient-packed soup brims with spinach's highly absorbable antioxidant vitamins and alkaline sea veggie minerals to keep you strong for life.

SERVES 1

2 cups (400 ml) filtered water

2 cups (400 ml) spinach leaves

½ cup (100 ml) peeled and chopped sweet onion

½ teaspoon (2.5 ml) dulse powder

½ teaspoon (2.5 ml) kelp powder

Pulse all the ingredients in a blender until smooth. Pour into a bowl, and enjoy.

Pumpkin Pleasure Soup

Filled with fiber and flavor, this savory soup's pumpkin seeds are high in zinc, magnesium, iron, protein, and essential fatty acids. Pumpkin seeds are known to promote men's fertility and help prevent prostate issues.

SERVES 1

½ cup (100 ml) pumpkin seeds, plus more for garnish

1 cup (200 ml) filtered water

1 cup (200 ml) pumpkin, peeled

2 pitted dates

Nama Shoyu or Tamari, to taste

Soak the pumpkin seeds in water for a few hours or overnight. Discard the liquid and pour the seeds into a blender with the filtered water. Add the pumpkin, dates, and Nama Shoyu and pulse. Pour into a bowl, garnish with additional pumpkin seeds, and serve.

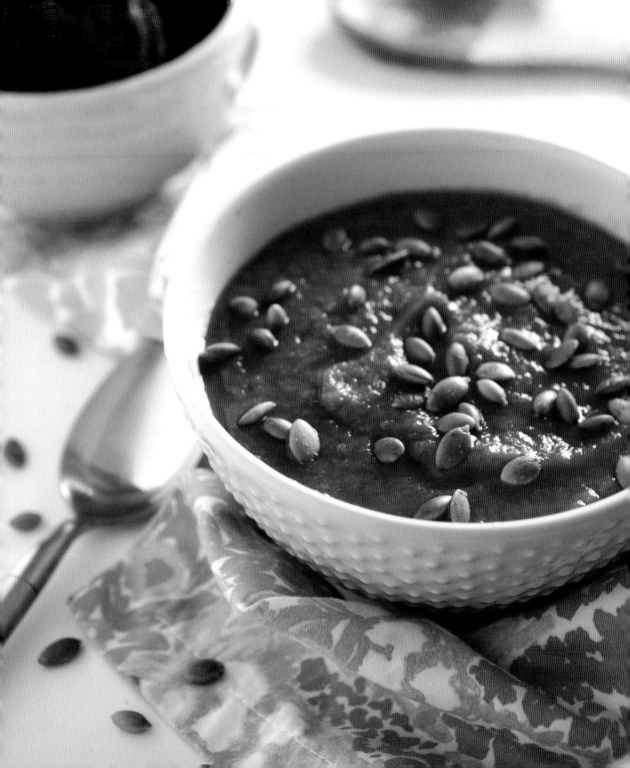

Cool Ginger Melon Soup

Revitalize yourself with this fresh, chilled soup. The melon of your choice, which is the basis of this soup, boosts your immune system and stabilizes your blood pressure.

SERVES 1

½ ripe melon (your choice of watermelon or any other melon in season), peeled, seeded, and chopped into chunks

Filtered water, as needed

½ inch (13 mm) fresh gingerroot

For garnish:

Handful fresh mint leaves

Place the melon, water, and gingerroot in a blender and pulse until smooth. Pour the soup into a bowl. Crumble several mint leaves to bring out the menthol and sprinkle atop the soup.

Broccoli and Leek Soup

Take the strain off an overstressed digestive system, and infuse your body with the liquid vitamins of the phytonutrient-rich cruciferous broccoli, the fertility-boosting healthy fats of the avocado, and the mild flavors of leek without feeling deprived.

SERVES 1

1 head broccoli, chopped into chunks (2 cups [400 ml]), plus a few more chunks for garnish

2 cups (400 ml) filtered water

3 medium leeks, chopped, plus 1 for garnish

1 avocado, peeled and pitted

1 tablespoon (15 ml) Nama Shoyu or Tamari

1 tablespoon (15 ml) fresh lemon juice

Place the broccoli, filtered water, leeks, avocado, Nama Shoyu, and lemon juice in a blender and blend. Pour into a bowl and top with a few small pieces of broccoli and a leek stalk.

Cream of Celery Soup

Stress hormone–reducing celery contains coumarins that help to lower blood pressure, reduce the risk of blood clots, and help regulate the body's water balance. Combine that with the blood sugar–balancing properties of zucchini, and you have yourself one heck of a detox soup!

SERVES 1

1½ cups (300 ml) chopped celery

2 cups (400 ml) filtered water

1 zucchini, cut into chunks

1 small garlic clove, peeled

1 tablespoon (15 ml) Nama Shoyu or Tamari

1 teaspoon (5 ml) ground fennel

For garnish:

1 celery stalk

Place the celery, water, zucchini, garlic, Namu Shoyu, and fennel in a blender and pulse until creamy. Pour into a bowl, and garnish with a celery stalk.

CHAPTER 11

ENTRÉES AND SIDES

THESE FOODIE-PLEASING ENTRÉES AND SIDES will tempt any taste buds and satisfy your hunger without that overstuffed feeling. They are delicious, filling, and the indisputable winner in nutrients over their heavily processed versions.

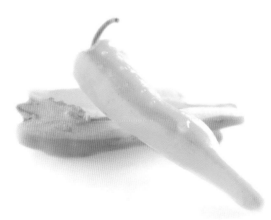

Cinco de Mayo Stuffed Peppers

This is one of my favorite recipes! It's absolutely delicious and easy to make. The secret is the cilantro, lime juice, and lime zest and the way these flavors blend with the rest of the veggies—yum! I could eat this every day. Sometimes I just make a big bowl of the stuffing and eat it all in one sitting!

SERVES 1

½ cup (100 ml) finely sliced carrots

1 orange bell pepper, cored, seeded, and chopped into bite-size pieces

1 bunch cilantro, chopped

½ cup (100 ml) bite-size broccoli florets

½ cup (100 ml) bite-size cauliflower florets

4 stalks scallions, finely sliced

½ cup (100 ml) fresh peas

Juice and zest from one lime (squeezed by hand), with zest reserved

1 teaspoon (5 ml) celery powder

2 red bell peppers, cored, seeded, and cut in half length-wise

Place the carrots, orange bell pepper, cilantro, broccoli and cauliflower florets, scallions, and peas in a large bowl, and mix well. Scatter the lime zest across the ingredients in the bowl, and pour in the lime juice. Sprinkle the celery powder throughout, and toss all the ingredients thoroughly. Stuff the mixture into the red pepper halves, and eat!

Chee-Z Cauliflower Mash

Sorry, Mom, but I don't miss your old-school mashed potatoes 'n' gravy after having this delicious, healthy version. And the best part? I can have seconds, guilt-free!

SERVES 1

3 cups (600 ml) chopped cauliflower florets

¼ cup (50 ml) pine nuts

Juice from one lemon (sqeezed by hand)

1 garlic clove, peeled

2 tablespoons (30 ml) filtered water

2 tablespoons (30 ml) nutritional yeast

2 teaspoons (10 ml) chopped chives

1 teaspoon (5 ml) fresh thyme

For garnish:

Crushed red pepper, to taste

Combine all the ingredients in a blender and pulse until smooth. (Or feel free to keep this dish a bit chunky, if you prefer!) Scoop into a bowl and add crushed red pepper.

NOTE: If you'd like to add more nutritional yeast for more chee-z flavor, go for it!

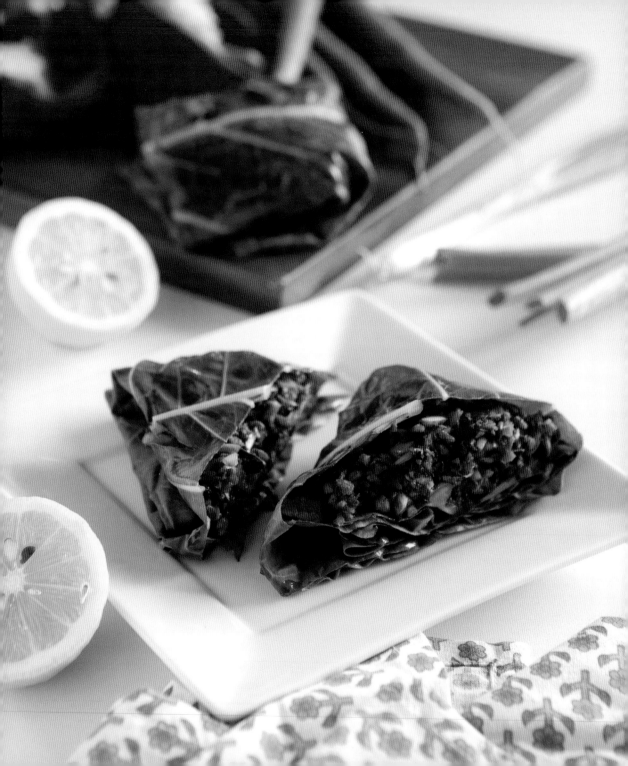

Collard-Wrapped Veggie Burger

This easy-to-make veggie burger beats the pants off those seemingly healthy store-bought frozen ones that actually have loads of unwanted chemicals and additives—check the box. But not in this version. What you see is what you get, and that's pure, clean, nutritional goodness!

SERVES 1

- 2 cups (400 ml) chopped mushrooms
- 1 red bell pepper, cored, seeded, and finely chopped
- 1 scallion, chopped
- 4 carrots, unpeeled and chopped
- ⅓ cup (67 ml) chopped fresh basil leaves
- 1 garlic clove, peeled and finely chopped
- 1 teaspoon (5 ml) dried oregano
- ½ teaspoon (2.5 ml) celery salt
- 2 collard greens

Prior to making this dish, chop and soak the mushrooms in Nama Shoyu for a few hours or overnight. Combine all the ingredients, except for the collard greens, in a bowl, and mix thoroughly. Form the mixture into thick, burger-size patties. Top each collard green leaf with a veggie patty, fold over the edges, and enjoy.

Hearts of Romaine Stuffed with Summer Squash Hummus

A delicious spin on traditional hummus and a great way to use up your summer harvest, this recipe uses yellow summer squash (or zucchini) and is a great source of manganese, found to alleviate monthly PMS mood swings and menstrual cramps.

SERVES 1

1 cup (200 ml) diced yellow summer squash (or zucchini)

½ cup (100 ml) raw tahini

Juice from one lemon (squeezed by hand)

2 garlic cloves, peeled

1 tablespoon (15 ml) Nama Shoyu or Tamari

1 teaspoon (5 ml) cumin powder

1 teaspoon (5 ml) turmeric powder or 2 inches (5 cm) turmeric root, grated

Black pepper, to taste

2 hearts of romaine leaves

Place all the ingredients except the black pepper and romaine leaves in a blender and pulse until smooth. Add black pepper to taste. Scoop the mixture into the hearts of romaine leaves.

Zucchini and Carrot Spaghetti with Sun-Dried Tomatoes and Red Pepper Sauce

Here's a guilt-free, nutrient-dense spaghetti that doesn't make you want to go take a nap, but actually gives you energy! And, no, there isn't any cooking with this spaghetti!

SERVES 1

Spaghetti:

1 zucchini

5 carrots

Sauce:

3 sun-dried tomatoes

½ cup (100 ml) filtered water

2 red bell peppers, cored, seeded, and chopped

1 date

1 bunch fresh basil

1 garlic clove, peeled

Juice from ½ lemon (squeezed by hand)

For garnish:

Oregano, to taste

Thyme, to taste

Dulse powder, to taste

Place the sun-dried tomatoes in a bowl of filtered water and soak for 20 minutes (this is separate from the filtered water on the ingredients list). Use a vegetable slicer or mandoline to slice the zucchini and carrots very finely or a spiral vegetable slicer and make a big plate of veggie spaghetti. Set aside.

Put all the ingredients for the sauce in a blender and pulse until velvety. Pour the sauce over the "spaghetti," and garnish with the spices and dulse powder.

Jicama Fries with Cayenne and Red Pepper Ketchup

I never had jicama before I tried jicama fries—and now I'm addicted. I'll bet you will be, too! Because commercial ketchup is so full of processed sugar, this no-sugar recipe was adapted from the Hippocrates Health Institute.

SERVES 1

Fries:

- 1 jicama
- Expeller-pressed extra-virgin olive oil
- Paprika, to taste
- Onion powder, to taste
- Ground flaxseed (optional)
- Psyllium husk powder (optional)
- Stevia (optional)

Ketchup:

- 1 red bell pepper, cored, seeded, and chopped
- ½ medium red onion, peeled
- ½ red beet
- Juice from ½ lemon (squeezed by hand)
- ¼ cup (100 ml) apple cider vinegar
- 1 tablespoon (15 ml) ground flaxseed, plus more for fries (optional)
- 1 teaspoon (5 ml) paprika
- 1 teaspoon (5 ml) celery powder
- 1 teaspoon (5 ml) garlic powder
- Filtered water, as needed
- Stevia, to taste

Slice the jicama into French fry-like wedges or use a potato slicer to cut it into wedges. Place the jicama fries in a container with a lid. Drizzle olive oil and sprinkle paprika and onion powder on the jicama wedges.

Close the lid and shake vigorously to distribute the oil and spices. You can add ground flaxseed or even psyllium husk powder to thicken, if desired, and stevia to sweeten.

Combine all the ketchup ingredients in a blender, and pulse, adding water as needed for desired consistency. Season and sweeten with stevia to taste.

Belgian Endive Stuffed with Green Pea Hummus

This recipe was given to me by a favorite doctor friend, Dr. Greg, who is also a chef, and boy did this combination produce a kick-butt creation that is not only good for you, but also contains some serious body and brain food.

SERVES 1

¼ cup (100 ml) walnuts

Juice from ½ lemon (squeezed by hand)

1 cup (200 ml) shelled fresh peas

1 garlic clove, peeled

½ avocado, peeled and pitted

1 teaspoon (5 ml) dulse powder

4 small Belgian endive leaves

For garnish:

A few walnut halves

Soak the walnuts in water for a few hours or overnight. Discard the liquid and put the walnuts in a blender; add the lemon juice, peas, garlic, avocado, and dulse to the blender and pulse until it reaches a hummuslike consistency. Pipe into Belgian endive leaves, and garnish with the walnut halves.

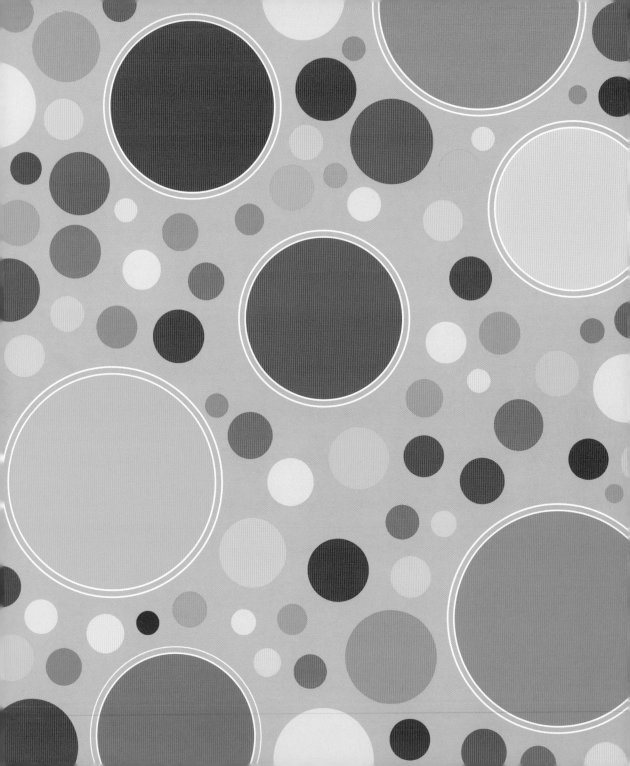

CHAPTER 12

SALADS AND DRESSINGS

NOT YOUR RUN-OF-THE-MILL SALADS, these recipes might just change your mind about the negative salad stereotypes out there.

● The Salads

All of you know how to make a salad. I've provided a few uncommon options to inspire you to think outside the box and maybe come up with some of your own. Utilize any of the oil-free rainbow dressings from pages 157–64 on the salads in this chapter.

● The Dressings

Dressing can make or break your salad, and it can just as easily make or break your weight. I never buy store-bought dressings

because of all the chemical additives and strange-sounding ingredients listed on the back of the bottle, but also because most of the seemingly healthy ones always use totally unhealthy oils, especially canola oil. All the dressings provided here are entirely oil-free and made instead with nourishing whole-food fats, not processed oils and no chemical preservatives. You can chill them for a few days in the refrigerator in an airtight jar, but it's best to make them fresh and use them immediately!

Rainbow Tricolor Spiral Salad

A salad without lettuce? Give this one a try. The sweetness of the carrots and the mild licorice taste of the fennel, complementing the delicate flavor of the squash, may leave you not wanting any dressing at all.

SERVES 1

5 carrots, unpeeled

1 yellow squash

1 bulb fennel

Use a vegetable slicer or mandolin to slice the carrots, squash, and fennel very finely, or a spiral vegetable slicer, and make a big bowl of spiral salad. Toss with your favorite Rainbow dressing.

Sea Veggie Salad

Sea veggies are jam-packed with trace minerals and some serious heavy metal–detoxing and bone-building properties. You definitely want this salad as a staple in your diet.

SERVES 1

Handful whole dulse
leaves

Handful whole kelp
leaves

Handful whole arame
leaves

Toss all the sea veggies in a big bowl with your favorite Rainbow dressing.

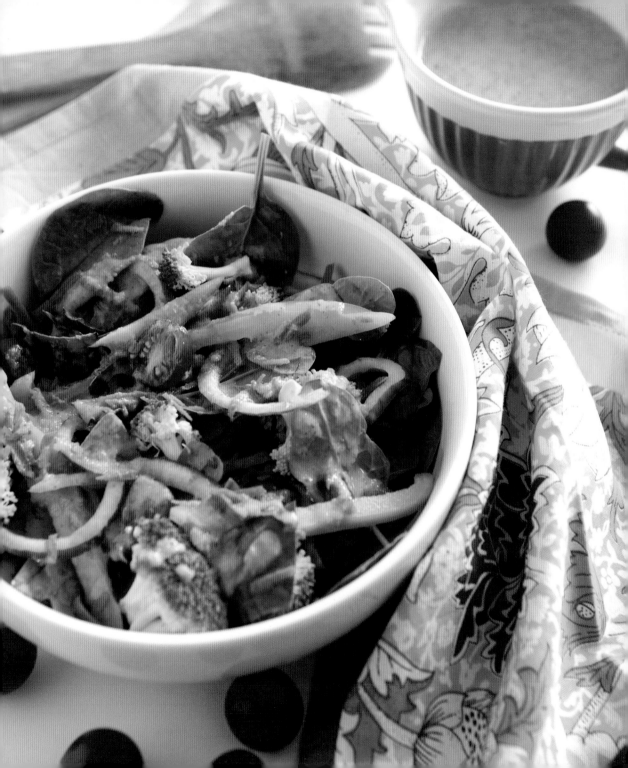

Rainbow Power Salad

We can't have a Rainbow Juice Cleanse book without a Rainbow salad! Every color, contrast, flavor, and texture of the rainbow is represented here, as are chlorophyll, magnesium, amino acids, and too many other goodies to name!

SERVES 1

1 head broccoli, cut into bite-size pieces

4 carrots, unpeeled and grated

1 yellow bell pepper, cored, seeded, and chopped

1 medium red onion, finely sliced

6 purple kale leaves, torn into pieces

¼ cup chopped walnuts

Handful spinach

Handful cherry tomatoes, sliced in half

Place all the ingredients in a big bowl, and top it off with a handful of halved cherry tomatoes and a delicious Rainbow salad dressing.

opposite: Rainbow Power Salad with Orange Pepper and Cilantro Dressing (page 157)

Queen of Quinoa Salad

Called the "mother of all grains" by the ancient Incans, quinoa (pronounced KEEN-wah) is a complete source of protein and a heart-healthy grain; it is known to help lower bad (LDL) cholesterol. This salad requires a little more prep time than most: Before you make the salad, you need to sprout the quinoa for one or two days in order to enhance its nutrient profile and rid it of its natural, bitter saponin coating to prevent potential stomach upset. Serve it as a main dish or as a hearty side dish plain, or toss it with any of the Rainbow salad dressings.

SERVES 1

1 cup quinoa

1 red bell pepper, cored, seeded, and finely chopped

1 carrot, finely chopped

1 bunch parsley, finely chopped

1 bunch mint, finely chopped

1 bunch scallions, finely chopped

1 stalk celery, finely chopped

½ cup (100 ml) sunflower seeds

Put the quinoa in a mason jar, and fill it with filtered water. Let it sit for about 6 hours or overnight. Strain the liquid off (you can use a mason jar sprouting lid). Fill the jar with filtered water again and strain it once again. Put the jar of soaked quinoa, lid-side down, in a bowl so the excess water can drain off. Every 6 hours (the timing doesn't have to be exact; do this when you remember, but not too much longer than 6 hours between rinses), rinse, drain, and set the jar back in the bowl for a total of 1 or 2 days, or until the first sprouts start to pop. Once you see this, place the jar in the fridge and make this recipe immediately or within a few days.

Place the quinoa and the rest of the ingredients in a big bowl and toss until well mixed.

Orange Pepper and Cilantro Dressing

Sweet and sassy and perfect on any salad! Since you are making it fresh, it's not pasteurized (a nutrient-destroying high heat) like most traditional salad dressings, so you are able to harness the full force of bioavailable nutrients. Loaded with vitamin C and phytonutrients like carotenoids, you are doing your body good!

SERVES 1

Juice from one large orange (squeezed by hand)

1 orange bell pepper, cored and seeded

½ bunch cilantro, chopped

1 cucumber, chopped into chunks

1 garlic clove, peeled

1 teaspoon (5 ml) white miso

Place the orange juice, pepper, cilantro, cucumber, garlic, and miso in a blender, and pulse well. Store in an airtight jar in the refrigerator.

Tomato Curry Cider Dressing

Light, healthy, and loaded with probiotics (the good-for-the-gut, healthy bacteria), this dressing is the perfect choice to top off any of the salads. The curry powder, with its combination of over twenty herbs and spices (depending on the brand)—including cayenne, red pepper, coriander, cumin, and turmeric— harnesses all the healing benefits and adds lots of nutrients.

SERVES 1

3 medium tomatoes, chopped into chunks

3 tablespoons (45 ml) apple cider vinegar

2 dates, pitted

1 garlic clove, peeled

1 teaspoon (5 ml) curry powder

Sea salt, to taste

Organic black pepper, to taste

Place all the ingredients in a blender, and pulse until creamy. Store in an airtight jar in the refrigerator.

Creamed Spinach Dill Dressing

This dressing is packed with good-for-you vitamins and antioxidants like vitamins K, A, B$_1$, B$_2$, B$_6$, C, E, and loaded with folate, magnesium, calcium, potassium, zinc, phosphorus, iron, selenium, and copper. The flavorful macadamia nuts provide monounsaturated fats known to help lower bad (LDL) cholesterol, as well as raise good (HDL) cholesterol.

SERVES 1

½ cup (100 ml)
   macadamia nuts

1 cup (200 ml) filtered
   water

2 cups (400 ml) spinach
   leaves

1 garlic clove, peeled

1 tablespoon (15 ml)
   Nama Shoyu or Tamari

1 tablespoon (15 ml)
   ground dill, plus more
   for garnish

Soak the macadamia nuts in distilled water for a few hours or overnight. Discard the liquid and place the nuts in a blender, along with the filtered water, spinach, garlic, Nama Shoyu, and ground dill, and pulse. Store in an airtight jar in the refrigerator and garnish with a dash of dill when serving.

Lemon Fennel Dressing

Indulge in the delicious, distinctive flavor of this health-boosting dressing. The alkalizing lemon and the detoxifying fennel provide bioavailable anti-inflammatory vitamin C, high blood-pressure fighting potassium, and loads of other nutrients, including the flavonoids, rutin, quercitin, and kaempferol.

SERVES 1

2 cups (400 ml) chopped fresh fennel

1 tablespoon (15 ml) ground fennel

1 cup (200 ml) filtered water (more or less, depending on desired consistency)

Juice from one lemon (squeezed by hand)

1 tablespoon (15 ml) Nama Shoyu or Tamari

Stevia, to taste

Place the fennel (chopped and ground), water, lemon juice, and Nama Shoyu in a blender, and pulse thoroughly. Add stevia, to taste. Store in an airtight jar in the refrigerator.

Green Goodness Dressing

My friend and colleague, Dr. Greg, knew what he was doing with this salad dressing! Research has shown absorption of the phytonutrients lycopene and beta-carotene increases significantly (up to 400 percent!) when avocado is added to a salad. Add to that the blood pressure lowering effects of the garlic and a heck of a lot of green via parsley, chives, and dill.

SERVES 1

1 avocado, peeled and pitted

½ cup (100 ml) fresh parsley, loosely packed

½ cup (100 ml) chopped fresh chives, loosely packed

½ cup (100 ml) fresh dill, loosely packed

½ cup (100 ml) filtered water (or more, as needed)

1 garlic clove, peeled

¾ teaspoon (4 ml) celery salt

Place all the ingredients in a blender, and pulse until smooth. Thin out the dressing with more water, if needed. Use immediately, or store in an airtight container in the refrigerator.

Cucumber Mint Dressing

Cucumbers and mint pair deliciously in this light and refreshing dressing—one of my favorites! It's loaded with nourishing phytonutrients from not only the green family, but also the white/tan and purple families as well. Savor away with this dressing and use it on any of the salads.

SERVES 1

1 cucumber, chopped into chunks

½ cup (100 ml) fresh mint leaves

1 garlic clove, peeled

Juice from ½ lime (squeezed by hand)

2 tablespoons (30 ml) peeled and finely chopped sweet onion

1 tablespoon (15 ml) dulse powder

Place all the ingredients in a blender, and pulse until creamy. Store in an airtight jar in the refrigerator.

Turmeric Tahini Ginger Dressing

Warm and super-nourishing, this dressing deserves a spot in your weekly diet. Anti-inflammatory, digestion-improving, and immune-system boosting, turmeric outperforms many prescription drugs in its effects against several chronic diseases from arthritis to cancer to Alzheimer's. Add it to any of the nutrient-dense salads or even use it as a dip.

SERVES 1

½ cup (100 ml) tahini

2 tablespoons (30 ml) apple cider vinegar

2 tablespoons (30 ml) Nama Shoyu or Tamari

2 tablespoons (30 ml) turmeric powder or 2-inch (5 cm) turmeric root, grated

1 teaspoon (5 ml) peeled and grated fresh gingerroot

¼ teaspoon (1.3 ml) black pepper

Filtered water, as needed

Combine all the ingredients in a small jar with a lid and shake vigorously until well mixed. Add water as needed for desired consistency. Store in an airtight jar in the refrigerator.

Yellow Pepper Vinaigrette Dressing

When you just can't take another balsamic vinaigrette, this is your go-to dressing. This healthy, oil-free alternative loads up on phytonutrients such as lutein, zeaxanthin, and beta-cryptoxanthin, as well as Vitamins C and K, many of the B vitamins, copper, manganese, magnesium, zinc, and omega-3 fatty acids from the flaxseed. Pour on the nutrients!

SERVES 1

1 yellow summer squash, chopped into chunks

1 yellow bell pepper, cored and seeded

¼ cup (50 ml) filtered water

Juice from ½ lemon (squeezed by hand)

1 tablespoon (15 ml) flaxseed

1 date, pitted

¼ teaspoon (1.3 ml) paprika

¼ teaspoon (1.3 ml) mustard powder

¼ teaspoon (1.3 ml) dried oregano

¼ teaspoon (1.3 ml) onion powder

¼ teaspoon (1.3 ml) dried thyme

Place all the ingredients in a blender, pulse well, and serve over your favorite salad. Store leftover dressing in an airtight jar in the refrigerator.

13

DESSERTS

SOME PEOPLE ARE INTRODUCED TO HEALTHY EATING through delectable, decadent, good-for-you desserts. I was one of those people. That day, I knew I would never feel deprived following a healthy-eating regimen. Once you discover your favorites, you may want to double-batch. Bring on the dessert!

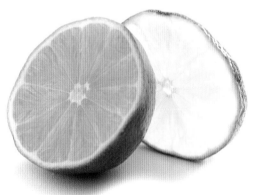

Mint Carob Chip Avocado Mousse

This is my all-time favorite snack for when I need a chocolate fix. The best part of all? There's no dairy! Use carob or cacao instead. And the avocado, you ask? Well, let's just say, you will be astounded by the taste.

SERVES 1

2 avocados, peeled and pitted

3 tablespoons (45 ml) unsweetened carob powder

5 fresh mint leaves, plus more for garnish

½ cup (50 ml) water or almond milk (optional depending on desired consistency)

Stevia, to taste (or a few dates, pitted and soaked)

For garnish:

Carob chips

Place all the ingredients in a blender, and pulse until smooth and thick. Add additional stevia as needed, and garnish with mint leaves and carob chips. Very important: Be sure not to eat it all before you give your family a chance to try it.

Strawberry Hazelnut Pudding

Strawberries blended in a creamy bed of hazelnut is sure to always be welcome at the table—if it ever makes it to the table! Try this recipe with different berries each time for delicious variations.

SERVES 1

1 cup (200 ml) hazelnuts

2 dates, pitted

½ cup (50 ml) coconut water

1 cup (200 ml) fresh strawberries

2 tablespoons (30 ml) unsweetened carob or carob powder

1 tablespoon (15 ml) alcohol-free vanilla extract or vanilla bean

For garnish:

Fresh mint leaves

Strawberries

Hazelnut halves, soaked

Soak the hazelnuts and dates in water for a few hours or overnight and then discard the liquid. Place the hazelnuts and dates in a blender, and pulse to combine. With the motor on low, drizzle in the coconut water, and drop in the strawberries one by one. Add the carob and vanilla, and turn up the motor, if needed. Add more coconut water or filtered water to achieve the desired thickness.

Scoop into a small bowl or ramekin, adorn with mint leaves, a few whole strawberries, and a few soaked hazelnut halves, and devour!

Blackberry Banana Split Ice Cream

Imagine a healthier soft-serve ice cream—it's totally doable and totally tantalizing. With ripe, frozen bananas to help lower blood pressure and keep the Big Pipe moving, just add blackberries (or the berries of your choice) for an antho-cyanin-phytonutrient blast.

SERVES 1

3 ripe bananas, peeled and chopped into chunks

2 cups (400 ml) fresh blackberries

Filtered water, as needed

For garnish:

Fresh banana slices

Fresh blackberries

Freeze the banana pieces and blackberries overnight or until firm. In a blender, pulse the bananas and blackberries with a little bit of water until a smooth, creamy consistency is reached. Garnish with banana slices and fresh blackberries before serving. Eat immediately, or let it set in the freezer for an hour.

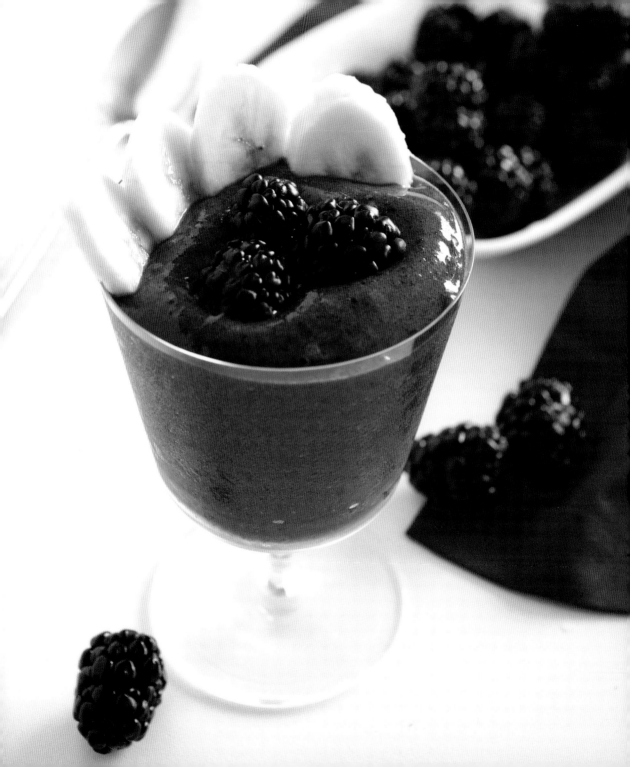

Mango Sorbet

This light, sweet, easy-to-make, high fructose, and corn syrup-free frozen dessert will delight your taste buds and your cells with vitamins C, A, and B_6; copper, potassium, and magnesium; and fiber.

SERVES 1

2 fresh mangos, peeled, pitted, and chopped into bite-size chunks

Juice from one lemon or lime (squeezed by hand)

Stevia, to taste (optional)

For garnish:

Fresh mint leaves

Freeze the mango pieces overnight or until frozen. Place the juice and frozen mango chunks in a blender. Pulse until well blended. Add stevia to taste. Once the desired consistency is reached, place the sorbet back in the freezer to firm up, about 15 minutes. Then garnish with some mint, and eat at once!

Pecan Pie Ice Cream

Nothing says Southern like pecan pie! Throw in some nondairy ice cream, and you've got yourself a scrumptious treat. And the cherry on top? This recipe's actually good for you!

SERVES 1

- 3 bananas, peeled and chopped into chunks
- 1 cup (200 ml) pecans, plus more for garnish
- 1 date, pitted and soaked
- 1 tablespoon (15 ml) alcohol-free vanilla extract or vanilla bean
- 1 teaspoon (5 ml) ground cinnamon
- 1 teaspoon (5 ml) ground nutmeg

Freeze the banana pieces for at least an hour or overnight. Soak the pecans and date in water for a few hours or overnight. Discard the liquid. Blend the bananas, pecans, and date in a blender. Add the vanilla extract, cinnamon, and nutmeg and pulse until a soft ice cream–like consistency is reached. Stir in some chopped pecans. Scoop into a bowl, and gorge!

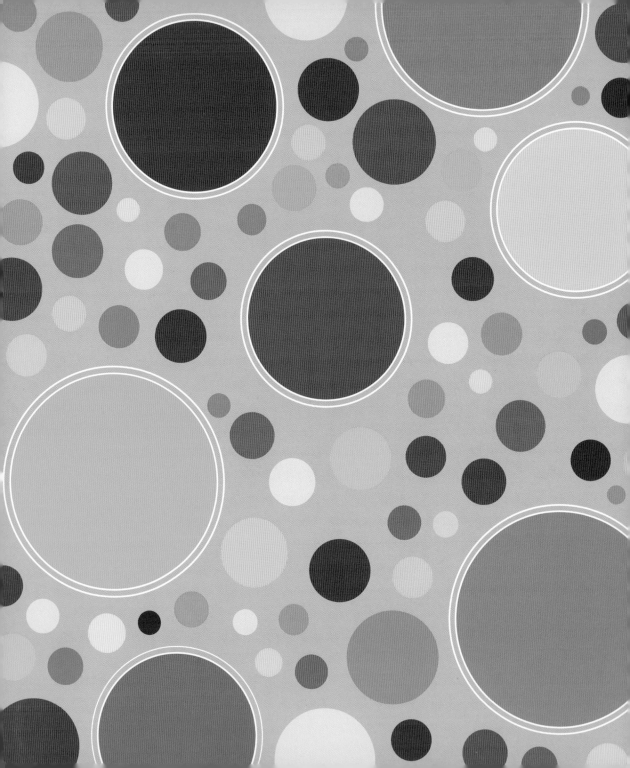

14

APPROVED FOODS

THE FOLLOWING LISTS feature the Rainbow Juice Cleanse approved foods you can eat during the warm-up phase and then bring on full force during the rev-up phase as well as the four days prior to and the four days after the all-juice seven-day Rainbow Juice Cleanse. They are easily digestible, highly nourishing, cleansing, raw (uncooked), and preferably organic foods that can become "regulars" in your new healthy Rainbow way of eating. You can find these foods at your local grocery or health food store. And don't forget to review the "Clean Fifteen" and the "Dirty Dozen" lists on page 47.

Note: Consult your physician if you have health challenges or are taking medications that have certain food restrictions.

DARK GREEN LEAFY VEGETABLES AND CRUCIFEROUS VEGGIES

Go overboard with these phytonutrient-packed foods! These are the staples of the Rainbow Juice Cleanse. Be sure to choose fresh, ripe, raw, organic, and unsweetened (except with stevia). Nothing frozen, canned, or bottled. Although there are about a thousand species of plants, here are some of the more traditional and easy-to-find options, loaded with alkaline minerals and easily absorbed amino acids—the building blocks of protein.

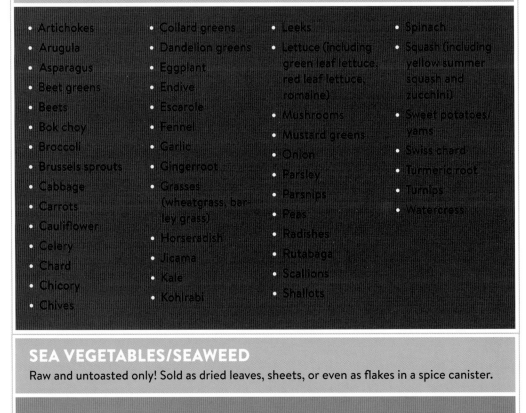

- Artichokes
- Arugula
- Asparagus
- Beet greens
- Beets
- Bok choy
- Broccoli
- Brussels sprouts
- Cabbage
- Carrots
- Cauliflower
- Celery
- Chard
- Chicory
- Chives
- Collard greens
- Dandelion greens
- Eggplant
- Endive
- Escarole
- Fennel
- Garlic
- Gingerroot
- Grasses (wheatgrass, barley grass)
- Horseradish
- Jicama
- Kale
- Kohlrabi
- Leeks
- Lettuce (including green leaf lettuce, red leaf lettuce, romaine)
- Mushrooms
- Mustard greens
- Onion
- Parsley
- Parsnips
- Peas
- Radishes
- Rutabaga
- Scallions
- Shallots
- Spinach
- Squash (including yellow summer squash and zucchini)
- Sweet potatoes/ yams
- Swiss chard
- Turmeric root
- Turnips
- Watercress

SEA VEGETABLES/SEAWEED

Raw and untoasted only! Sold as dried leaves, sheets, or even as flakes in a spice canister.

- Alaria/wakame
- Arame
- Dulse
- Hijiki
- Kelp
- Kombu
- Nori

SPROUTS

Jam-packed with nutrients and very easy to sprout at home. Add sprouts to your juices, salads, sandwiches, or anywhere you can squeeze them in! Here are just a few.

- Adzuki bean sprouts
- Barley
- Broccoli sprouts
- Buckwheat
- Cabbage sprouts
- Chickpea/ garbanzo bean sprouts
- Lentil sprouts
- Mung bean sprouts
- Pea sprouts
- Quinoa sprouts
- Radish sprouts
- Sunflower sprouts
- Wheatberries and wheatgrass sprouts
- Wild rice sprouts

HERBS AND SPICES

These are some of the most highly pesticide-sprayed plants, so be sure to buy organic!

- Basil
- Black pepper
- Cardamom
- Cayenne pepper
- Celery powder
- Chili powder
- Chives
- Cilantro
- Cinnamon
- Cloves
- Coriander
- Cumin
- Curry
- Dill
- Fennel
- Garlic cloves and garlic powder
- Gingerroot and ground ginger powder
- Horseradish
- Italian herb mix
- Marjoram
- Mint
- Mustard
- Nutmeg
- Oregano
- Paprika
- Parsley
- Parsley flakes
- Pizza seasonings (oregano, majoram, basil, garlic powder)
- Rosemary
- Sage
- Thyme
- Tumeric root and turmeric powder
- Vanilla bean (whole pod or powdered)

FRUIT

Fresh, ripe, raw, unsweetened, and organic. Nothing frozen, canned, or bottled. Fruit has higher concentrations of fructose sugar, so restrict your intake—especially in your juice or all-fruit fruit juices—if you're trying to lose weight, or if you have diabetes, cancer, or yeast or bacterial infections. Eat more greens!

- Apples
- Apricots
- Bananas
- Blackberries
- Blueberries
- Carob
- Cherries
- Cranberries
- Dates
- Figs
- Grapefruit
- Grapes (red)
- Jackfruit
- Kiwi
- Loquat
- Mango
- Melon
- Mulberries
- Nectarines
- Oranges
- Papaya
- Passion fruit
- Peaches
- Pears
- Persimmons
- Pineapples
- Plums
- Pomegranates
- Prickly pear/panini/cactus fruit
- Raspberries
- Strawberries
- Tangerines
- Watermelon and its rind

NONSWEET FRUIT

- Avocados
- Bell peppers (red, orange, yellow)
- Coconuts
- Cucumbers
- Eggplant
- Lemons and their rind
- Limes
- Okra
- Pumpkins
- Squash
- Tomatoes
- Zucchini

FATTY FRUIT

Don't go overboard, but don't be afraid of these fruits loaded with good-for-you fats.

- Avocados
- Durian
- Olives

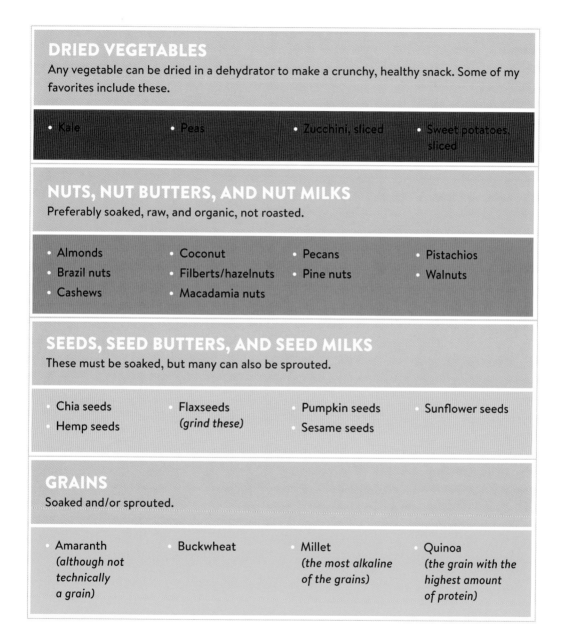

DRIED VEGETABLES

Any vegetable can be dried in a dehydrator to make a crunchy, healthy snack. Some of my favorites include these.

- Kale
- Peas
- Zucchini, sliced
- Sweet potatoes, sliced

NUTS, NUT BUTTERS, AND NUT MILKS

Preferably soaked, raw, and organic, not roasted.

- Almonds
- Brazil nuts
- Cashews
- Coconut
- Filberts/hazelnuts
- Macadamia nuts
- Pecans
- Pine nuts
- Pistachios
- Walnuts

SEEDS, SEED BUTTERS, AND SEED MILKS

These must be soaked, but many can also be sprouted.

- Chia seeds
- Hemp seeds
- Flaxseeds *(grind these)*
- Pumpkin seeds
- Sesame seeds
- Sunflower seeds

GRAINS

Soaked and/or sprouted.

- Amaranth *(although not technically a grain)*
- Buckwheat
- Millet *(the most alkaline of the grains)*
- Quinoa *(the grain with the highest amount of protein)*

BEANS AND LEGUMES (see sprouts)

FATS AND OILS

I'm not a fan of bottled oils, but if you must, use these, and only use coconut oil when you're heating something up. Choose organic whenever possible, and always choose cold/expeller-pressed/virgin oils, meaning the oil is from the first press, not the leftover oil at the bottom of the barrel.

- Almond oil
- Avocado oil
- Coconut meat/ pulp
- Coconut oil/ butter (*the room temperature determines its consistency*)
- Flaxseed oil
- Hempseed oil
- Olive oil
- Sesame oil
- Sunflower oil
- Walnut oil

FERMENTED FOODS

These foods rank high in good-for-you intestinal bacteria, aid in digestion, and are rich in enzymes and full of flavor.

- Apple cider vinegar (*I prefer Bragg's raw, organic, unpasteurized*)
- Kimchi/raw sauerkraut (*not fermented with vinegar!*)
- Miso, tempeh, natto
- Nama Shoyu (*raw, unpasteurized soy sauce; contains wheat*)
- Nutritional yeast (*adds a cheesy flavor and substantial nutrients; is not bread yeast*)
- Probiotic drinks
- Tamari (*unpasteurized soy sauce; usually wheat/ gluten-free*)

SUPERFOODS

These are the foods of the future—loaded with amino acids, vitamins, minerals, essential fatty acids, and chlorophyll. Work these into your daily lifestyle, and watch your health soar.

- AFA/Aphanizom-enon flos-aquae (freshwater blue-green algae; E3Live brand)
- Chlorella (high-protein green algae)
- Green powders (dehydrated cereal grasses and veggies)
- Spirulina (high-protein blue-green algae)
- Sprouts (see the Sprouts section in this chapter, page 175)
- Wheatgrass juice

SOY

Consume fermented soy products only!

- Miso
- Nama Shoyu
- Natto
- Tamari
- Tempeh

LIQUIDS

- Cucumber water (add a few slices of cucumber to a glass of water, or even add cucumber juice)
- Filtered water only, no straight tap water!
- Fresh-made organic veggie juices and veggie smoothies
- Lemon water (you can also add a touch of cayenne pepper)
- Naturally decaf-feinated, organic, herbal teas (peppermint, ginger, etc.)
- Probiotic/fermented drinks
- Young coconut water

OTHER

- Carob powder and carob chips
- Chickpea miso
- Manna breads (*yeast-free, sprouted breads*)
- Plant-based protein powders (*pea, cranberry, almond, hemp*)
- Raw cereals, granolas, and crackers
- Raw desserts (*pudding, ice cream, etc.; see recipes on pages 165–71*)
- Raw entrées (*burgers, spaghetti, etc.; see recipes on pages 141–49*)
- Raw milks and protein shakes (*see recipes on pages 125–29*)
- Raw nut and seed butters
- Raw nut and seed cheeses
- Raw protein bars (*look for "raw" on the label*)
- Raw sauces, dips, and spreads (*guacamole, salsa, pesto hummus, etc.; see recipes on pages 141–49*)
- Raw trail mix
- Sea salt (*use sparingly; I prefer sea veggies for natural sodium and that "salty" flavor*)
- Seed crackers (*flax, chia*)
- Sprouted breads and tortillas (*look for "sprouted" on the label; usually baked, so you can make it yourself in a dehydrator if you want it raw*)
- Stevia (*the best sweetener*)
- Tahini (*sesame seed spread*)
- Vanilla extract (*alcohol-free*)
- Young coconut meat

REFERENCES

"America's Phytonutrient Report." *Exponent for Nutrilite* (February 1, 2010).

Anderson, C., Rayalam, S. "Phytochemicals and Adipogenesis." *Biofactors* 36, no. 6 (November–December 2010): 415–422.

Avena, N., Pedro, R. "Excessive Sugar Intake." *Neuroscience and Biobehavorial Reviews* 32, no. 1 (2008): 20–39.

Billiot, M., DC. "Sugar and Your Immune System: Dr. Linus Pauling's Forgotten Research." www.alternativehealthatlanta.com (accessed August 18, 2014).

Brand-Miller, J., Foster-Powell, K. *The New Glucose Revolution Low GI Guide to Losing Weight.* Cambridge, Mass.: Da Capo Press, 2003.

Bravo, K. "How the Sugar Industry Is Using Big Tobacco Tactics to Downplay the Danger of Your Sweet Tooth" (July 20, 2014), www.takepart.com (accessed August 18, 2014).

Chopra, D., M.D. "All Great Changes Are Preceded by Chaos." www.soulpancake.com (accessed September, 15, 2014)

Clement, B., PhD, NMD, LN. *Food Is Medicine: The Scientific Evidence*, vol. 1. Summertown, Tenn.: Hippocrates Publications, 2012.

Corliss, J. "Eating Too Much Added Sugar Increases the Risk of Dying with Heart Disease." *Harvard Health Blog* (February, 6, 2014), www.health.harvard.edu (accessed August 18, 2014).

Cousens, G., MD. *There Is a Cure for Diabetes.* Berkeley, Calif.: North Atlantic Books, 2008.

Environmental Working Group. "The Shopper's Guide to Pesticides in Produce" (2014), www.ewg.org (accessed August 18, 2014).

Fed Up. Dir. Stephanie Soechtig. Dis. Radius-TWC. 2014. DVD.

Gates, D., Sahelian, R. *The Stevia Cookbook: Cooking with Nature's Calorie-Free Sweetener.* New York, Penguin Putnam, Inc., 1999.

Hyman, M., MD. "Are Your Hormones Making You Miserable?" (November 17, 2011), www.huffingtonpost.com (accessed August 18, 2014).

"Isaac Newton Explained the Colors of the Rainbow" (January 25, 1975), www.lookandlearn.com (accessed August 18, 2014).

Lawoyin, S., Sismilich, S. "Bone Mineral Content in Patients with Calcium Urolithiasis." *Metabolism* 28 (1979): 1250–54.

"Leading Causes of Death." Centers for Disease Control and Prevention. (October 10, 2010), www.cdc.gov (accessed August 18, 2014).

Mercola, J., DO. "Fructose: This Additive Commonly Used in Food Feeds Cancer Cells, Triggers Weight Gain, and Promotes Premature Aging" (April 20, 2010), www.mercola.com (accessed August 18, 2014).

"National Diabetes Statistics Report." American Diabetes Association. (2014), www.diabetes.org (accessed August 18, 2014).

Sterline, J. "America's Wacky Fair Foods." (July 31, 2011), www.foodandwine.com (accessed August 18, 2014).

"Sugars and Sweeteners." USDA Economic Research Services. (May 26, 2012), www.ers.usdda.gov (accessed August 18, 2014).

"Sugar Intake Guidelines." World Health Organization. (March 5, 2014), www.who.int (accessed August 18, 2014).

"The Sweet Life and What It Costs Us." Face the Facts USA. George Washington University. (December 21, 2012), www.facethefactsusa.org (accessed August 18, 2014).

"The Tomato: Fruit or Vegetable?" www.tomato-dirt.com (accessed August 18, 2014).

Tsuda, T. "Regulation of Adipocyte Function by Anthocyanins: Possibility of Preventing the Metabolic Syndrome." *Journal of Agricultural and Food Chemistry* 56, no. 3 (2008): 642–46.

"28 New Foods at Minnesota State Fair in 2014." (June 25, 2014), www.myfoxtwincities.com (accessed August 18, 2014).

WEB RESOURCES

RainbowJuiceCleanse.com

If you liked this book, you will love the website! Sign up for the newsletter, and get even more rainbow phytonutrient information and cutting-edge research on cleansing and supercharging your diet and your life!

TheDrGinger.com

Log on here for more information about Dr. Ginger and her future appearances. Sign up for her free "Healthy Steps with Dr. Ginger" newsletter, too.

FatFuneralDetox.com

Join like-minded individuals interested in becoming and staying healthy, with access to even more weight loss advice, cutting-edge scientific information, and product recommendations, such as homeopathic formulas; plant-based, heavy metal–free protein powders; whole food–based supplements; detox products like zeolite; and superfoods like spirulina and chlorella.

HippocratesInstitute.org

On the official website for Hippocrates Health Institute—voted the number one medical spa in the world by *Spa* magazine—you will find articles on nutrition, healing, growing sprouts, disease, and many other topics. Be sure to sign up to receive the institute's free quarterly magazine, *Healing Our World*. You will want to read every issue cover to cover.

InfraredSauna.com

Clearlight Infrared Saunas are the best carbon/ceramic infrared saunas I have found. They feature a patent-pending, virtually EMF-free heating technology and are made with eco-certified sustainable woods. Mention "Dr. Ginger," and get a discount on your order.

RawFor30Days.com

This is the official website for *Simply Raw: Reversing Diabetes in 30 Days*, the documentary that chronicles six people with diabetes and their journey to reverse their diabetes through food, not medicine.

Ewg.org

The Environmental Working Group website is an excellent resource for consumer health information and consumer guides on everything from nontoxic cleaning supplies to pesticides in produce to safe sunscreens.

TheChinaStudy.com

One of the best resources for the whole food, plant-based diet movement from T. Colin Campbell's *New York Times* bestselling book, *The China Study* is a must-read for anyone who wants to learn the truth about nutrition.

Pcrm.org

The Physicians Committee for Responsible Medicine is a nonprofit organization that promotes preventive medicine and alternatives to animal research. This site provides great resources on cancer, diabetes, and other reports, as well as surveys and clinical research studies.

KrisCarr.com

A former student—gone wild! With her fun and sassy style, you will gain great insight from a brave and determined woman, who didn't let her cancer diagnosis take her down.

NaturalNews.com

A science-based natural health advocacy website, founded by Mike Adams, "The Health Ranger," and a great daily source to hear the latest news you won't read on mainstream news sites concerning holistic health, nutritional therapies, environmental health, and many other important topics.

ForksOverKnives.com

An empowering website inspired by the 2011 documentary of the same name that is helping to change the way the world understands nutrition and its direct impact on disease.

Vegan-Up.com

My friend, chef Terry Botel, really gets it when it comes to making the absolute healthiest dishes—and I love his gift for creating delicious meals using the pulp from his daily juices!

VeganBodyBuilding.com

If there is one person who knows how to stay healthy and lean, and build big, strong muscle on a plant-based diet (the kind of foods and juices in this book), it's Robert Cheeke. Check out his site to take your physique to the next level in weight training.

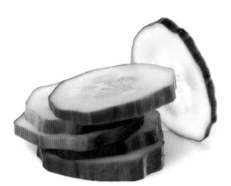

ACKNOWLEDGMENTS

FIRST AND FOREMOST, I give my unbounded love and gratitude to God.

Thank-you to everyone at Running Press for your extraordinary vision and your unswerving standards of excellence. To the incredible group that worked so hard to help make this book a reality, I've enjoyed the privilege of being part of your elite team!

A great BIG thanks and bear hug to my editor and guardian angel, Jordana Tusman, whose superb editorial and organizational skills were critical in helping me pull all of my information together and breathe life into my manuscript. I humbly bow to your insights. You made this book an absolute pleasure to write!

To my genius book designer, Susan Van Horn, for the beautiful colors and the clean design. You truly turned my manuscript into a visual masterpiece. I can't wait to see the expression on my mother's face when she sees it. Thank-you! Thank-you!

To my publicists, Allison Devlin and Seta Zink. You found so many opportunities for me it made my head spin! Thank-you for all your energy and attention and for believing in what I have to say. You two are true pros!

My deepest appreciation to photographer extraordinaire, Allan Penn, for the beautiful, colorful, delicious photos that made me want to go back and make the recipes again as soon as I saw them. I wish I had you on hand every time I whipped up a juice or a recipe!

I would also like to pay a very special tribute to my God-sent literary agent, Holly Schmidt, for coming up with the perfect title in an inspired, creative moment and for "getting" my concepts and my message. You have guided me from a writer to an author. Thank-you for all your encouragement and support and for believing in me. I am forever grateful.

I am deeply appreciative to everyone who made this book possible through your loving support, recipes, scholarly contributions, inspiration, and/or insight. You all helped in little ways that made a big difference, including:

Julie Abernathy, Mike Alden, Rona and Jeff Alexander, Christy and Doug Allen, Robert G. Allen, Rob Anderson, Ken Bailey, Bruce and Karen Banker, Jack Barnathan, Jason Beach, Richard Beckman, Jonas Beel, Phil Benninger, Deleon Best, Ron Bistolfo, Jane, Bruce, Sophie, and Alex Bolen, Ron Blakeney, Shaun Blick, Ward Bond, Cameron Bott, Jennifer Brown, Deanna and Blake Burns, T. Colin Campbell, Kris Carr, Christopher Carroll, Phillip Carrol, Pete Cervoni, Linda Chaé, Ian Chandler, Alex and Dan Cohn, Robert Cheeke, Conor Chibnall, Leighanne Chilmaid, Bob Choat, Holly Clark, Brian and Anna Marie Clement, Jay Comer, Fred Cooper, Stephanie Danburg, Lisa Davis, Cheryl Dearmon, Aaron Decker, Andy Decker, Pat and Jim Decker, Allyson Dennis, Donna Detwiler, Aisha Dew, Cathy Dewar, Gerald Dillard, Mike Dimayuga, Doug and Florence Dodd, Christine Dolbeare,

Kelly Donahue, Andrea Donsky, Chris and Judy Doyle, Raleigh Duncan, Mary Luther-Eggleston, Luz Evangelista, Joel Fuhrman, Mark Fields, Marla Finn, Molly First, Stephen First, Cassie and Tim Frankland, Eliza and Scott Friedman, Scott Gaddy, Wendy and Fred Galle, Ann and Dink Gardner, Clay Hair and Woodson Gardner, Bobby Genovese, Stone and Carter Hair, Donna Gates, Ashleigh Gass, Clif Gentile, Kevin Gilbert, Robert Goldman, Rene and Ron Goff, Vincent and Valerie Green, Shane and Bonnie Greene, Holly Gregg, Susan Hamilton, Gary Hanger, List Hannig, Harry Harden, Bill Harloff, Becky and Tom Heitman, Danielle and Paul Hayter, Andy Hope, Pat Horton, Melanie Householder, Mark Hyman, Jan and Charles Ison, Kerry Jacobson, Tommy Johnson Sr., Tyler Jones, Lisa Kapantais, Andy and Caroline Kaps, Alan Kauffman, Olivia Kauffman, Lisa and Todd Keiser, Amy Kleinklaus Lee, Josh Koepp, Greg Kuldanek, Jennifer Lambert, Deanna Latson, Jennifer and Lee Lein, Seth Leitman, Jay Lipoff, Cindy Long, Sikung Grandmaster Lowe, Terry Lyles, Bernard and Maria McCue, Dave McDaniels, Debbie Miller, Kathy Miller, Constance Mollick, Leilani Munter,

Beth Nash, Ross and Debra Nash, Margaret Osborne, Jim O'Brien, Melissa O'Toole, Marvin Pantangco, Lynette Marie Pate, Casie Petersen, Tonya Phillips, Kent Piskin, Jay Poonkasem, Sue Pyle, Jenifer Quinn-Wilson, Janet Randolph, Bruce Ressen, Pat Rogers, Dawn and Tom Rofrano, Joe Rovitto, Todd and Ashley Rowland, Tim and Laura Sales, Chad Sarno, Andrew Saul, Angelia Savage, Rebecca Schieber, Linda Naismith Schultz , Matt Sharkey, Lori Shemek, James Sherwood, Kevin and Sam Sorbo, Scott, Karrie, Richmond and Keagan Southall, Bruton Smith, John St. Augustine, Jennifer and Brandon Stites, Peyton, Ryan, Carson and Kellen Stites, Mike Stone, Ray Strand, Steve and Myrna Swartz, Angel Teems, Riley Timmer, Dara Torres, Reginia Turner, Lenore Vassil, Jesse Vista, Dave and Laura Vroman, Don and Tina Vroman, Claudia Waddell, Jessica Walkington, Amy Wilkinson, Wellons Wilkinson, Brian Wilson, Don and Lori Wallace, Susan and Tim Wipperman, Mark Wilson, Lance Wood, Jeff Yates, Wenhan Zhang, Eric Zayes, Bobby Zeitler, Matt Zerebney, and Kristen and DJ Zorn.

Thank you all!

INDEX

NOTE: Page references in *italics* indicate photographs.